Moral Dilemmas in Medicine

# Moral Dilemmas in Medicine

## A COURSEBOOK IN ETHICS FOR DOCTORS AND NURSES

### ALASTAIR V. CAMPBELL
M.A., B.D., Th.D.

*Lecturer in Christian Ethics, University of Edinburgh. Lecturer in Ethics, RCN Institute of Advanced Nursing Education (Scotland)*

Foreword by Professor A. S. Duncan

Second Edition

CHURCHILL LIVINGSTONE
EDINBURGH LONDON AND NEW YORK
1975

CHURCHILL LIVINGSTONE
Medical Division of Longman Group Limited

Distributed in the United States of America by
Longman Inc., 72 Fifth Avenue, New York,
N.Y. 10011 and by associated companies,
branches and representatives throughout the
world.

First edition 1972
Reprinted 1974
Second edition 1975

ISBN 0 443 01286 5


Library of Congress Cataloging in Publication Data
Campbell, Alastair V
    Moral dilemmas in medicine.

    Includes bibliographies and index.
    1.  Medical ethics.  I.  Title.
[DNLM:  1.  Ethics, Medical.  W50 C187m]
R724.C33  1975        174 .2            75-7819

# Foreword

By A. S. DUNCAN

D.S.C., F.R.C.S.E., F.R.C.P.E., F.R.C.O.G.

*Professor of Medical Education and Executive Dean of the Faculty of Medicine, University of Edinburgh*

Scientific progress, technological advances and a permissive attitude to behaviour bring benefits to society but they also introduce difficult dilemmas. Hardly a day passes without the newspapers featuring examples of such problems as Dr Campbell discusses in this book. The problems affect all of us and each of us has to make up his or her mind about the issue involved. No longer can the decisions be made by the health professions alone with the patient or relative as a silent acquiescent. The members of the public must understand the issues and participate in decisions which affect them as individuals or which affect the priorities and attitudes of the community in general.

Doctors and nurses will, of course, be expected to give a lead in these matters, and the public will often still prefer that the decision be made on their behalf. By their greater experience, workers in the health field should be able to offer guidance, but many young doctors and nurses, on completion of their training, feel they have received little teaching on moral or ethical issues. Curricula have become so loaded with the very scientific and technical matters which lead to the dilemmas that little time is left for thought as to the dilemmas themselves.

Many teachers in schools of medicine and nursing do raise these issues with their students, but lack the background of training and reading of the theories of moral philosophy, and so are only able to give a rather superficial view, often biased by personal experience. The early specialisation at school means that students of medicine sorely lack the broader education which should form a proper base for thinking on moral issues.

If doctors and nurses lack background knowledge of moral theories, how much more does the general public. This book is written primarily for the health professions, but the general reader will find in it much food for thought, and will learn to appreciate the issues which underlie the decisions in which he, as a patient or a citizen, will be called upon to play a part. The book will, I believe, fill a very real gap in education—a gap which at the present time is only partly bridged by extra-curricular discussion in groups and societies.

Dr Campbell, in his preface, expresses some misgivings that, as a medical layman, he should be discussing decisions of which he has no personal experience. I believe that the view from the side lines can be more objective, and Dr Campbell, with his training in moral philosophy, his special experience in the health field and his interest as an adviser of students, is particularly well fitted to write on the moral dilemmas which face us all. He is careful not to impose his own views or to suggest that for every problem there is a right and wrong answer. Rather does he guide us through the different theories and provide us with the background material and thinking which will allow each of us to make up our minds with intelligent comprehension rather than with emotional bias on the basis of isolated or limited personal experience.

# Preface to the Second Edition

Since publication of the first edition of this book two and a half years ago interest in medical ethics has increased dramatically. The founding of the *Journal of Medical Ethics* by the London based Society for the Study of Medical Ethics has provided a new organ for international and interdisciplinary discussion of the issues. Two American institutes—the Kennedy Centre for Bioethics, Georgetown and the Hastings Centre, Hastings-on-Hudson, N.Y.—have sponsored multidisciplinary research and publication in the field. Judging from the attention paid to medico-moral problems by the news media, public interest is also very great, and it is noticable that the over-simplifications of earlier years are now largely avoided. It seems that the public participation in medical decisions, to which Professor Duncan refers in his foreword, is now becoming a reality, at a surprisingly technical level.

Revising a book is both gratifying and frustrating. My intention to write a useful textbook for doctors and nurses has been realised beyond my own expectations and in view of this I have not altered the expositions of the classical theories of ethics. I have however extensively revised the section dealing with current problems. In addition to up-dating references, I have made more explicit the relationships between the problems and the alternative ethical theories. But the frustration of a reviser comes from a feeling of 'all or nothing'. Perhaps this is why, in the concluding section, there are hints of a new beginning.

For advice about this revision I am grateful to Rev.

Werner Becher, Miss Margaret Halsey, Rev. David Lyall, Rev. Stewart Macgregor and, especially, Dr Robin Gill.

A.V.C.

Edinburgh,
February, 1975

# Preface to the First Edition

This book has been written with the concerns of doctors and nurses primarily in mind, but I hope that it may also prove of interest to members of other professions, and indeed to anyone who feels a sense of responsibility for health and welfare in modern society. My intention is to provide a short introduction to some of the major theories of moral philosophy and to relate these to contemporary moral problems in medical care. I have organised the material under a set of broad topic headings and have listed references to other literature in moral philosophy and medical ethics. In this way I hope to have laid the foundations of a short course in ethical theory in relation to medicine, which may be used both by medical and nursing educators and by individuals interested in teaching themselves more about the subject.

While writing this book I have experienced two kinds of misgiving. On the one hand I have been conscious of the fact that as a medical layman I am discussing decisions of which I have no personal experience: on the other hand, as an interpreter of the technicalities of ethics to philosophical laymen, I am aware of the healthy suspicion which professional philosophers have of those who try to simplify and popularise complex philosophical arguments. I have put aside my misgivings, however, because I feel that there is a high value in communication between the ethical theoretician and the medical decision-maker whatever the risk of intellectual blunders involved.

Several people have assisted me during the planning and

composition of this book. (Factual inaccuracies and errors of judgment, which remain despite advice, are of course entirely my responsibility.) All the examples of moral dilemmas used to illustrate the theoretical points have been supplied by doctors and nurses out of their own clinical experience. I am particularly grateful to students and former students of mine in the Royal College of Nursing, Edinburgh for providing enough material to fill several books on the subject. At various stages of writing I have received detailed advice from Miss A. T. Altschul, Professor J. C. Blackie, Professor R. H. Girdwood, Miss M. C. N. Lamb, Rev. T. S. McGregor, Dr P. R. Myerscough and Professor Sir Michael Woodruff. I am especially indebted to Professor A. S. Duncan, Executive Dean of the Faculty of Medicine, Edinburgh University, who, in addition to writing the Foreword, has provided stimulation, encouragement and correction throughout the period of writing.

The completion of the typescript was made possible by the accurate and tireless secretarial work of Mrs Jacquie Young. It was also greatly aided by the kindness of the minister of Durisdeer Kirk, the Rev. J. W. Scott, who made available as a study a quiet and beautiful room, in what were formerly the ducal retiring rooms of the kirk.

My greatest debt is to my wife and children. For many months they tolerated the vagueness and impracticality of the juggler with ethical abstractions.

ALASTAIR V. CAMPBELL.

Edinburgh. April, 1972.

# Contents

# CHAPTER ONE

# Moral Dilemmas and Ethical Theories

A patient in the ward in which I worked was visited by the surgeon in the evening after his operation. The surgeon asked how the patient was, and being told that he appeared to be suffering severe pain prescribed five milligrams of diamorphine injected intramuscularly. The patient was given the injection, but had a restless sleep and clearly was still in pain. When the surgeon returned to the ward in the morning and was told of the patient's condition he ordered an increase of dosage to *fifty* milligrams. Knowing that an increase of this magnitude was almost certainly lethal, I questioned the surgeon's instruction. He appeared rather taken aback by my questioning, but explained that while operating the previous day he had found that the patient's abdomen was riddled with carcinoma.... I went to the ward clinic to draw up the injection knowing full well that it would kill the patient. I hesitated to think what I was doing. To end the patient's life was against all my upbringing, my nursing experience and my religious conviction. But could I refuse? I had been in the hospital only a week after qualifying as a registered mental nurse and this was one of my first difficult situations. If I refused to give the injection that might be the end of my career in general nursing. What was I to do?

This description of a situation encountered by a newly qualified nurse conveys what it is like to be faced by a moral dilemma. Not all situations are as dramatic as this one. The unusual situation of a doctor passing on such an instruction to a nurse, newly qualified and unsure of his position, sharpened the dilemma. But more and more frequently difficult personal decisions have to be taken by doctors and nurses involved in the complexities of modern medicine, many of them concerned with the choice between life and death or between life which is worth living and life which is hardly preferable to death. This book explores some of these dilemmas, relating them to theories of ethics put forward by moral philosophers at different periods of history. We shall try first to understand what are the essential features of the moral dilemmas occurring in medicine and then what theories of ethics have to do with them.

## Moral Dilemmas

In a dilemma one is faced with two alternative choices, neither of which seems a satisfactory solution to the problem. The nurse drawing the lethal injection believed that he had to choose between killing the patient and jeopardising his own future. (This was how he saw the situation, even although in fact a nurse's right to refuse to carry out such an order would normally be respected.) It seemed that he had a simple choice between self-interest and respect for the life of another human being, the right, if not the easiest decision being to refuse to carry out the surgeon's orders. But in the nurse's mind there was also uncertainty about whether it was more humane to preserve the patient's life or to put a final end to his pain. This meant that, for the sake of keeping his own conscience clear, he might be causing more suffering to the patient, and possibly to the patient's relatives, in addition to putting in danger the security of his own family. It looked as though, whichever decision he took, he might be acting wrongly.

Dilemmas like this arise in situations of ambiguity

and uncertainty, when it is difficult to predict the consequences of one's actions, and when the general principles upon which one normally relies either offer no help or seem to contradict one another. Which action would cause the least unhappiness all round? Was it more important to preserve life or to prevent pain? There seemed to be no answers to the nurse's questions from the set of convictions about right and wrong with which he had operated up to that point.

Frequently the full force of the moral dilemmas involved in medicine is avoided by a less drastic approach to problems than that described in the example. Many doctors would not make so direct an attack on human life as that involved in the sudden increase in dosage of morphine. But a gradual increase in the dosage, necessitated by the patient's increased tolerance to the drug, will often have the same life-shortening effect in the long-term. Thus a choice, though one not so obvious to the outsider, has still in fact to be made.

There are many situations of apparent moral dilemma for which solutions can be found. In the case of terminal illness great advances have now been made in the development of methods of controlling pain which do not endanger the life of the patient (Twycross, 1975). Had these been available at the time, the surgeon and the nurse would not have had to make any choice between maintaining life and preventing suffering. As the range of techniques and treatments available to doctors increases many of the old problems of choice between unsatisfactory alternatives have been solved. Unfortunately new techniques also bring fresh moral dilemmas. The development of organ transplantation, for example, has removed some of the problems connected with the care of patients suffering from kidney or heart disorders, only to replace them with new dilemmas concerning the permission of donors and the life-expectancy of recipients.

Moral dilemmas will continue to occur in medicine so long as choices have to be made which involve putting one set of values against another. Such decisions have to be distinguished from the many important *clinical* decisions which also must be taken by doctors. These decisions may often present dilemmas too, but the resolution of such problems is dependent solely on the doctor's knowledge, experience and intuitive abilities in medical matters. All these factors are certainly helpful to the person with a moral dilemma in medical practice, but they are not in themselves sufficient to unravel the moral conflict, because in the moral dilemma a different kind of decision has to be made. Thus, it is important to distinguish the dilemma in choice of *treatments* faced by the medical team caring for a person with advanced carcinoma, and the kind of choice made by the surgeon in our opening example. In the former situation choices have to be made between, say, the alternatives of surgery, radiotherapy and simply supportive and palliative measures. The dilemma has to be resolved according to skilled diagnostic assessments concerned with which treatment will be the more beneficial to this particular patient. But in the latter situation the decision taken was that it was better to hasten the patient's death. In making that choice the surgeon had abandoned the concept of treatment and chosen an action which he regarded as an act of mercy to a fellow human being. No amount of *medical* expertise could help either the surgeon or the nurse involved to know whether the decision was a right one.

The kind of dilemmas we are concentrating on, then, are those which raise fundamental questions about right and wrong actions in that part of human interaction which is concerned with the treatment of sickness and the promotion of health in our societies. That is what we mean by *moral dilemmas in medicine*. Dilemmas of this type have always been evident in the practice of medicine. It is significant that as far back as the 5th Century B.C. when medicine was in its infancy, the school of the physician Hippocrates adopted an oath which guided their moral decisions. This oath has remained the basis of codes of medical ethics right up to modern times (*see* Guthrie, 1957; Gelfand, 1968). The formulation of an oath or a code, however, does not do away with the moral choices, as we shall shortly illustrate. In fact the opposite often appears to be the case: the more concerned the profession of medicine and nursing have become about the formulation of codes of ethics the more they have become aware of the complexity of the moral problems facing them. When is termination of pregnancy justified? Should badly deformed children be kept alive? What are the right priorities in medical treatment and research? How 'officiously should we strive' to keep dying patients alive? All these questions and many others are being debated by doctors, nurses and the lay public. At the centre of the debates are a set of choices which have to be made, and about which there are deep disagreements and uncertainties.

## Ethical Theories

Faced with the kind of dilemmas we have been describing, people vary widely in reaction. Many people seek to handle situations of uncertainty by elevating their personal convictions to the status of inerrant and all-embracing rules, which must apply to every situation, whatever its complexities and ambiguities. Others try to reduce all moral dilemmas to questions of technical skill. Both these reactions are commonly found among doctors and nurses, many of whom may feel that there is little to be argued about in medical ethics, either because they do not themselves see any moral ambiguities in their professional practice or because they consider all the decisions taken to be purely matters of clinical judgment.

The activity known as moral philosophy or ethics is another way of reacting to moral uncertainty. Moral philosophy, like other forms of philosophy (such as the philosophy of science or the philosophy of artistic values), is characterised by the spirit of radical enquiry. Its approach is summed up in a saying of the Greek philosopher Socrates: 'The unexamined life is not worth living' (Plato, *Apology*, 38a). Philosophers are constantly questioning the common sense ideas which people have about truth, goodness and beauty. Thus Socrates went around Athens asking people what they meant when they used words like 'virtue' or 'justice'. His interrogation was so persistent and so unsettling that he was eventually tried on charges of blasphemy and corrupting the youth, and condemned to death. This persistence in looking for clarification in the use of concepts has been a constantly recurring emphasis in Western philosophy. Many systems of thought have been elaborated during the historical development of the subject, but none has been allowed to remain unexamined. No sooner has one school of philosophy achieved the position of the accepted way of understanding things, than a fresh set of questions has been asked which undermine its certainty.

Clearly then moral philosophy does not attempt to 'solve' moral dilemmas. Often, because of the constant questioning of every assumption, it may seem to make matters worse!

What it attempts to do is to provide a rational framework for understanding the complexities of moral judgment. The ethical theorist tries to clarify the meaning of words like 'good', 'ought' and 'right', which are part of everyone's daily vocabulary, yet used in many conflicting and ambiguous senses. In looking for clarification he is also trying to formulate a coherent basis for the moral judgments which these words express. As we shall see in subsequent chapters of this book, many kinds of explanations have been offered in the history of ethics. Some writers have related words like 'good' and 'ought' to the psychological state of the person using them—seeing them as expressions of his desire for happiness or of his benevolent feelings toward others; other theorists have looked for a basis for judgment in the 'objective world' outside the particular individual—such as in the social benefit resulting from actions or in the extent to which actions are in conformity with universal laws of morality; others again have been concerned to understand the character of the decision-making which seems to lie at the centre of moral judgments. The diversity of ethical theories is in fact about as wide as the diversity of ways of understanding the relationship between man and his environment.

The word 'ethics' itself is frequently a cause of confusion and misunderstanding. It will be used in this book to mean that area of philosophical theory which is concerned with understanding the nature of moral judgment. Defined in this way it means the same as the longer term 'moral philosophy'. It must be clearly distinguished from other activities often called 'ethics' in everyday speech. The most common confusion is between 'ethics' and 'morals'. Most people use these words interchangeably, especially in their adjectival form 'ethical' and 'moral'. The Greek and Latin words from which the English words derive do in fact mean roughly the same thing—'that which is customary, or generally accepted'—but for the purposes of describing the philosophical study of morality a distinction has to be made. Thus, 'ethics' is used to describe the formal study of morality, while 'morals' is used to describe the particular actions, beliefs, attitudes and codes of rules which characterise different societies, groups, and individuals. In other words 'morals' is the word for those phenomena which are studied by ethics.

If this distinction is understood it will be obvious that ethics in this sense is not concerned to provide any form of specific *moral guidance* such as rules for right behaviour or lists of virtues and vices. That is the purpose of particular systems of morality, often drawn up in the form of written codes of morality and often associated with a particular set of religious beliefs. (The Law of Moses or the teachings of Mahomet are good examples of such codes.) The ethical theorist, whatever his personal convictions, has to take up an uncommitted attitude to all systems of morality. His function is not one of moral guidance but one of objective analysis.

A second area of confusion is that between ethics and other disciplines which investigate moral beliefs and behaviour. Historians, anthropologists, sociologists and psychologists frequently study the moral attitudes of individuals, groups and whole cultures. Like the ethical theorist they attempt to approach the subject in a detached and analytical manner, but they ask *different kinds of questions*, according to the theoretical framework of their discipline. An anthropologist like Margaret Mead, for example, is interested in the rules for behaviour taught to children and adolescents in primitive cultures. In her perceptive studies of young people in Samoa and New Guinea she conveys the atmosphere of the culture and its differences in approach from that of Western societies (Mead, 1928; 1930). Such information is of great interest to the ethical theorist, but he would then go on to ask more abstract questions. He would wonder what the implication of the differences in moral rules about say, sexual behaviour between Samoan and American or European cultures have for the idea that there can be universal rules of morality which apply to all cultures. Thus, ethics is constantly trying to move from *description of the particular situation* to the *analysis of universal principles and concepts*. This means that ethics is a different kind of study from the history, sociology or psychology or morals, although the findings of these descriptive studies of morality are of considerable relevance to the ethical theorist.

## Ethics in Relation to Moral Dilemmas in Medicine

Now that something of the abstract, analytical, uncommitted approach of ethics has been outlined, the obvious question arises: of what possible use is it to relate the practical and compelling moral dilemmas which confront doctors and nurses to such a generalised, non-practical set of questions? In a sense this question can only be answered by reading some or all of the subsequent chapters of this book, where the value of the juxtaposition is put to the test. If the independent status of the discipline of ethics (and of its parent discipline philosophy) is to be maintained, there is no simple answer to the question. The values upon which the activity of philosophising are based are those of lucidity, coherence and comprehensiveness. Ethical theories are not formulated with a view to their relevance to particular situations or their practical value for certain individuals. Often, because of its totally abstract and generalised nature, people either inside or outside the discipline of philosophy have suspected that 'the Emperor has no clothes'—that because philosophical theories say nothing specific, they say nothing at all—they are comprehensively, coherently and lucidly naked! That suspicion should perhaps always be in the mind of the student of ethics, but it may be an overstatement of the case. All ethical theories return at one point or another to particular situations, in order to exemplify the concepts being discussed or to discover the practical implications of a principle being formulated. It is this movement back and forth between the particular and the general, which gives the subject a potential value for the contemporary dilemmas of those working in medicine. The intellectual discipline which such an activity imposes may assist the individual in an indirect way when faced with difficult moral choices. The analytical attitude which it teaches prevents reliance on unquestioned assumptions, or on uncritical reactions to particular situations, as escape routes from thinking through the complexities of adequate medical care.

We can illustrate the relationship between ethics and moral dilemmas in medicine in a general way by referring to the basic moral codes which guide the professional conduct of doctors and nurses. The medical profession has regarded the Oath of Hippocrates as the basis for judgments of ethical and unethical conduct. A modernised version of the Oath entitled *The Geneva Convention Code of Medical Ethics* was adopted by the World Medical Association in 1949. The International Council of Nurses formally adopted a code in 1953 (revised in 1965) under the title: *The International Code of Nursing Ethics*. The full texts of these Codes will be found in the Appendix, but for the present we are interested only in the fundamental principles of right conduct in medical and nursing practice which they enunciate. Both Codes take as their guiding principle the concept of *service to mankind*. The doctor solemnly pledges himself to consecrate his life to the service of humanity. The Nursing Code states that service to mankind is 'the primary function of nurses and the reason for the existence of the nursing profession'. Closely allied to the concept of service to humanity is the concept of *respect for human life*. The Medical Code states this in the following terms: 'I will maintain the utmost respect for human life from the time of conception; even under threat'. The Nursing Code adopts 'the essential freedoms of mankind' and 'the preservation of human life' as its fundamental concepts.

It may seem perverse to quarrel with these as adequate statements of basic principles, for, it is very unlikely that they could be improved upon as summaries of the primary aims of medicine and nursing. Yet in an important respect they are quite inadequate: they fail to provide answers to the really difficult moral problems in medicine. (This is a weakness which, as we shall argue later, *any* formal code is bound to have, although some philosophers would dispute this.) For example, the concept of respect for human life from the time of conception does not prevent doctors from terminating pregnancies under certain conditions, though what these conditions are, the code does not tell us. Clearly, the term 'respect' needs further investigation. The ambiguities are still more clear in the nursing code, the first clause of which reads as follows: 'The fundamental responsibility of the nurse is threefold: to conserve life, to alleviate suffering and to promote health'. There are many situations in which these three responsibilities cannot all be met. When a patient who has massive brain damage and is being kept alive by artificial means contracts an infection of the lungs, the decision whether or not to treat the infection with antibiotics involves a choice between conserving life and promoting health. The machine might be of much greater use elsewhere, whilst to continue the apparently hopeless condition of the patient might seem far from promoting anyone's health, not even his. Although the decision to treat or not to treat is a medical not a nursing one, both professions in such a situation are closely involved in the implications of trying to respect life without necessarily prolonging biological functioning at all costs. Appeal to the 'rule book' of either profession provides no answers. The same kind of difficulties arise in the conflict between the alleviation of suffering and the conservation of life. (For example, in the decision whether or not to keep severely deformed neonates alive); and in the conflict between the alleviation of suffering and the promotion of health. (For example, the use of treatments which may alter the personality of the patient, such as pre-frontal leucotomy.)

What is lacking in the codes of professional ethics is a searching analysis of the apparently simple terms out of which they are constructed—terms like 'respect', 'life', 'suffering' and 'health'. Admittedly, had an attempt been made to analyse these, the codes would probably never have been written, for, their meaning depends on many arguable assumptions about the nature and value of human existence. All that a profession can be expected to do is to provide some generalised statements in everyday language and leave it to the good sense and good will of its practitioners to deal with the ambiguous situations. But the ethical theorist *is* concerned to examine terms like 'respect', 'humanity', 'suffering' (and its converse 'happiness'). Thus it is precisely at the point at which the codes cease to be helpful that the debates between rival ethical theories become interesting and relevant. Does the notion of the 'voice of conscience' provide a basis for the concept of 'respect for life'? Can there be an inclusive system of moral law which will apply to all men as the basic laws of humanity? Could we measure the rightness of actions according to the amount of happiness they cause or the amount of pain they prevent? These are the questions which will concern us in the chapters which follow as we attempt to interrelate ethical theories and concrete problems of medical and nursing care.

## REFERENCES

Gelfand, M. (1968). *Philosophy and Ethics of Medicine*. Edinburgh: Livingstone.

Guthrie, D. J. (1957). The Hippocratic Oath. In *Medical Ethics*, p. 154ff. Ed. Davidson, M. London: Lloyd-Luke.

Mead, M. (1928). *Coming of Age in Samoa*. (Penguin Books edition, 1969.) London: Penguin.

Mead, M. (1930). *Growing Up in New Guinea*. (Penguin Books edition, 1970.) London: Penguin.

Saunders, C. (1972). The care of the dying patient and his family. *Contact*, **38** supplement, 12-18.

Twycross, R. G. (1975). The use of narcotic analgesics in terminal illness. *Journal of Medical Ethics*, Vol. 1, No. 1 (March), 10-17.

# CHAPTER TWO

# The Individual Conscience

Most people, if asked what they would do in a situation of moral uncertainty, are likely to refer to the notion of the guidance of conscience. Conscience is thought of as a kind of inner voice or authority warning you against wrong-doing and creating remorse when the warnings have been disregarded. The authority of conscience is frequently re-inforced by belief in a Divine Will underlying the moral principles which the individual conscience commands. If no religious belief is held, a person may still invest his conscience with considerable authority, seeing it as the articulation of the fundamental human values to which he is committed.

The idea of conscience as a guide to right behaviour is clearly of importance in the practice of the medical and nursing professions. Although these professions have be-come virtually completely divorced from religious institu-tions (in Western industrialised societies at least), they still carry strong vocational emphasis deriving from their his-torical associations with religious Orders and monastic foundations. The atmosphere of high dedication to humanitarian ideals is conveyed by the ethical codes of both professions; and other statements of firm personal commitment abound in the 'lore' passed on to new genera-tions of students. Examples of these are the often quoted *Prayer of a Physician* ascribed to the twelfth-century Jewish physician Maimonides:

Endow me with strength of heart and mind so that both may be ever ready to serve the rich and the poor, the good and the wicked, friend and enemy—and may I never see in the patient anything else but a fellow creature in pain.

and the Florence Nightingale Pledge for Nurses which contains the promises:

I solemnly pledge myself before God and in the presence of this assembly to pass my life in purity and to practise my profession faithfully ... With loyalty will I endeavour to aid the physician in his work, and devote myself to the welfare of those committed to my care.

To point to these emphases in the statements of ideals of the two professions, is not to make any assessment of how far these ideals are in fact adhered to in present day practice. We could only answer such a question by a thorough empirical survey of the attitudes and clinical practice of modern doctors and nurses. However, even without such evidence, it seems reasonable to assume that 'following conscience' will be the most common way in which doctors and nurses seek to solve the moral dilemmas which they encounter. We shall, therefore, begin our exploration of ethical theories by looking at the kind of theory which gives conscience or 'moral sense' a central place in the analysis of moral judgment.

## Conscience Theories

When we begin to look a little more closely at the common sense notion of conscience, a number of difficulties begin to show themselves immediately. We may use phrases like 'the small voice of conscience' or 'the inner light of reason' to express what we mean, but we are hardly likely to take such phrases literally. They are just metaphors we use to convey the immediacy of the feeling of obligation which conscience imposes on us. *Is* there any way behind the metaphors we use? If not literally a voice or a light, what kind of faculty is conscience? How do we know that the guidance it gives us is correct? And how is it that some people seem to be more influenced by their consciences than others? The attempt to answer questions of this kind results in the framing of theories of conscience. We shall look at two examples of such theories.

One way of describing the operation of conscience is to compare it to the artistic or aesthetic sense. This view of conscience is called the *Moral Sense Theory* and its best known exponent is **Anthony Ashley, Earl of Shaftesbury** (1671–1713). Shaftesbury argued that men have the capacity to distinguish between good and evil just as they can distinguish the beautiful from the ugly:

No sooner are actions viewed, no sooner the human affections and passions discerned ... than straight an inward eye distinguishes and sees the fair and the shapely, the amiable and the admirable apart from the deformed, the foul, the odious or the despicable. (*Characteristics of Men, Manners, Opinions, Times*, II, 415.)

Shaftesbury was aware of course that some men have greater sensibility than others in these matters, but he believed that it was possible to cultivate the moral sense just as it was possible to develop artistic appreciation. A few men might be *connoisseurs* of moral value, but any one had the capacity to sense the basic distinctions between good and bad actions.

The attractiveness of the moral sense theory is that it conjures up something of the subtlety of conscience-following behaviour. Both the immediacy and the complexity of moral judgment are conveyed by the comparison with appreciation of works of art. But Shaftesbury's theory has at least one serious deficiency, which we may outline briefly now, preparing to return to it at greater length, after exposition of a second theory of conscience. The theory does not take *variation in moral judgment* sufficiently into account. People's 'intuitions' about right and wrong often conflict sharply. A case in point would be differing views of the morality of abortion, some people seeing no moral objection to aborting a fetus for 'social' reasons, others finding such an act totally repugnant. Of course we can find the same diversity of viewpoint in questions of artistic merit also. Some people find great beauty in the music of, say, Schoenberg or Bartok—to others it is sheer cacophony. In the case of *artistic* judgment, however, we are able to accept diversity of opinion. We may argue a little about the merits of contemporary music, explaining the theory underlying it, but faced still with someone who finds no pleasure in it, we would be content with the explanation that in artistic questions tastes vary. The same does *not* hold in the majority of arguments about moral questions. In these cases variation in judgment is a much more important matter. We would not be prepared to say, for example, that the limits imposed on clinical experimentation or the type of nursing care given to the mentally subnormal are matters for individual taste or preference. Thus the analogy with artistic sense seems to break down. The fact of disagreement about moral questions demands a more thorough discussion of the *reasons* we might give for judging one action right and another wrong. The appeal to an immediate feeling of rightness does not take us far enough.

A more elaborate theory of conscience was given by **Joseph Butler** (1692–1752). This theory contained within it a psychologicial analysis, of which the following is a brief outline, phrased in modern psychological language as well as Butler's own terminology: Butler was concerned to demonstrate that having and obeying a conscience was part of what it meant to be a human being. Without the faculty of conscience human nature lacked coherence and balance; and equally integrity of personality demanded that the conscience was in harmony with the individual's basic needs and with his ability to reason. Butler compared the human personality to a mechanism like a watch, whose different parts have no use in isolation from their relationship to one another. Only when we have seen the interlocking of balances, gears and spring, do we appreciate the function of each individual part. Similarly, Butler argued, we cannot understand conscience by isolating it from those other factors in human beings which move them to action.

To modern eyes, Butler's psychological analysis of human motivation is perhaps rather too simple. He divides motives to action into three main types: 'particular passions and affections'; 'rational calculating principles'; and 'conscience', which he defined as: '... the faculty which surveys, approves, or disapproves the several affections of our mind and actions of our lives, being that by which men are a *law to themselves* ... (*Sermons*, 2, 14). The 'particular passions' include a wide range of motivations: basic drives like hunger or sex, emotional reactions like anger or fear; character traits like shyness or aggressiveness. Butler makes no attempt at distinction between these diverse elements since he is interested in the characteristics they have in common. The common feature is their *particularity*, that is to say they do not refer beyond themselves to the general aims and intentions of the person who experiences them but push for outlet or satisfaction in the present moment. The phrase 'blind impulses' seems best to convey what Butler was describing.

Human action, however, is not merely the result of impulsive reactions to situations—it is also characterised by forward planning on the basis of past experience. Therefore in the fully functioning personality, the *rational calculating principles* come into play. These principles control the impulses according to reasoned assessments of the long-term consequences of different actions. Such consequences can be assessed in terms of the future welfare of oneself or in terms of the future welfare of others who will be affected by the action. The calculation of one's own long-term happiness Butler called the Principle of Cool Self Love; the calculation of happiness of others, the Principle of Benevolence. These two principles provide the channels for direction of the particular passions in ways that will ensure the avoidance of the destructiveness and unhappiness which the immediate gratification of the impulse of the moment may bring.

An illustration related to medical care may help to clarify this part of Butler's analysis of human motivation. A natural reaction to the human suffering encountered in hospitals is an overwhelming feeling of pity or sympathy for particular patients, which can make it extremely difficult to offer a consistent pattern of professional, medical or nursing care. Junior nursing and medical students soon learn that they must not become 'over-involved' with patients if they are going to be able to continue in their chosen careers. Yet, however 'professional' a student learns to become, the essential emotional component of involvement with the patient's suffering must remain also. This mixture of rational and emotional elements is precisely what Butler is talking about when he speaks of the interdependence of passions and rational principles. Both because of the student's own career plans (Cool Self Love) and because of what will be genuinely beneficial to the patients (Benevolence), the impulses have to be controlled and directed, but not cancelled out, by a training in scientific assessment of medical conditions.

Butler believed that for the most part the channelling of the impulses by our ability to predict and plan the outcomes of action would be all that was necessary for a harmonious and happy existence. He did not see any violent opposition between the principles of Cool Self Love and Benevolence, since for the most part our own happiness was most easily found by seeking the happiness of others. There would be occasions, however, when an appeal beyond the assessment of long-term happiness would be necessary. This would be needed when a choice between the happiness of self and the happiness of others had to be made, or when a calculation of consequences gave no clear indication of the right decision to be taken. In such instances the final source of motivation and control should be *conscience*. Conscience goes beyond the prediction of consequences of actions to the assigning of moral value to them. It is a faculty of judging between right and wrong, by which the fully balanced individual exercises final control over decisions. There is no appeal beyond conscience since what it commands is not merely that which is desired, or that which is advantageous, but that which is *right*. To act in conformity to our true human nature is to act ultimately under the authority of the right. Therefore conscience holds a natural superiority over the other driving forces in our personality.

Before going on to criticise Butler's account of conscience, we must avoid a common misunderstanding of what he is saying. In claiming absolute authority for the faculty of conscience, he is not suggesting that all men *do* in fact act in accordance with their consciences. This would be tantamount to saying that no moral wrongs are ever committed, and Butler is well aware that many are. All that he is saying is that when we disobey our consciences we are destroying the natural balance of our personalities. To be truly human is to be a conscience-following individual, because conscience has an over-riding claim over us. But most people at one time or another, Butler realises, fall short of this ideal humanity.

The following frank and detailed assessment of the pressures to stifle moral sensitivity in a situation of mal-treatment of patients, which has been written by a senior nursing administrator, provides an excellent illustration of the kind of breakdown of the natural superiority of conscience' which would be interpreted by Butler as a dehumanisation of the individuals involved:

In my earlier days in psychiatric nursing I was at times perturbed at the lack of compassion to patients shown by certain members of the nursing staff. This resulted in a personal dilemma. I knew that incidents of this kind should be reported, but to do this would mean to stand alone against the 'closed ranks' of my colleagues. I was not at all sure how the nursing administration would react, the experience of others having shown that silence was often the best policy. I was faced with difficulties to do with witnesses of the incidents, loyalties to colleagues, future career prospects and even personal safety. I had seen things happen in the past and had no illusions about what might be done to the 'non-conformist'.

So far as I can see the trouble in such a situation is that one tends not to respond immediately to one's sense that wrong is being done. Thus the dictates of conscience become less clear and are eventually stifled to the extent that self interest takes precedence over patient interest. In theory the patient comes first, but in practice this is not necessarily so.

Despite the fact that it was written over two centuries ago, Butler's description of the various components in moral decision-making still provides an illuminating set of categories for discussing moral dilemmas. His aim was to stay as close as possible to the plain man's understanding of his own experience, and it seems that in pointing to the contrast between impulsive and planned action, the interdependence of self-interest and consideration of others, and the authoritative claim which conscience makes for its pronouncements, he has reflected everyday experience very well. Although the science of psychology has expanded rapidly over the past few decades, it would be difficult to find a system of moral psychology which improves on Butler for elegance of description (*see* Wright, 1971, for a survey of more modern systems).

From the point of view of ethical analysis, however, Butler's theory solves few, if any, problems. The crux of the difficulty lies in his confident assumption that the individual's conscience will give a clear and inerrant answer to all moral dilemmas. Certainly, in a rather unhelpful logical sense, his analysis is flawless: If conscience is that faculty in man which always guides him into right action, then conscience ought always to be obeyed. It is logically correct to state that man ought to do that which, in order to be truly human, he ought to do! The trouble is that the argument moves round in a circle and therefore is totally uninteresting. The question we are really concerned with is one which Butler never seems to ask: *Does conscience always guide the individual correctly?* And how do we know that it does?

## Conflict of Conscience

We find that we are back at the fundamental objection which had to be brought against Shaftesbury's Moral Sense theory. If the consciences of individuals tell them different things, who is to say which conscience is correct? We shall now explore this question in more detail by looking at some examples of conflict of conscience in hospital care. Although some of the examples chosen are ones in which there is conflict of opinion between medical and nursing staff, this is, of course, by no means the only kind of disagreement which can occur. Frequently doctors will disagree strongly among themselves over questions of conscience and the same is true of nurses. However, the dilemma is perhaps even greater where one person is in the position of carrying clinical responsibility for the decision, whilst the other's primary role is to carry out instructions. The examples below may be seen as illustrations of the potential conflict contained in clause seven of the *International Code of Nursing Ethics*: 'The nurse is under an obligation to carry out the physician's orders intelligently and loyally and to refuse to participate in unethical procedures'. The problem is who defines 'unethical', if the doctor and nurse disagree.

The first example is illustrative of the kind of problem which the British Abortion Act of 1967 has created. (Curiously, the fact that this Act contained within it a 'conscience clause', seems to provoke as much as solve problems.)

Nurses are placed in a considerable dilemma when asked to carry out treatment by medical staff which is contrary to what they believe to be right. Should students who have strong moral convictions in this area be asked to train in gynaecological wards where their principles cannot be taken fully into account if the work of the unit is to continue? In practice it is now very difficult to dissociate yourself completely from terminations of pregnancy. Formerly, there was a clearer demarcation between directly helping in theatre and being indirectly involved in post-operative care. Now with the advent of intravenous Pitocin drips the night nurse may be counting the drops and changing the rate without realising that this is the latest way of being directly involved. Some students decide that, since, whatever *they* do, the work will proceed, they ought to take their share of it. The situation is full of difficulties both for the staff and for the medical and nursing administration. The former have to find ways of coming to terms with their scruples about abortion: the latter to meet the twin demands of providing an adequate service for the patient and supporting those daily involved with the patient.

We can see immediately in this example the problem of the individual conscience in situations where complex social responsibilities are in operation. The conscience of the individual nurse may tell her that abortion, although at present legally sanctioned, is morally wrong, but this alone does not solve the conflict of obligations with which she is faced. The situation is similar to that of the person whose conscience is opposed to all forms of war and who may consider withholding part or all of his tax payments in order not to support expenditure on armaments. Complete opting out is legally possible for the nurse opposed to abortion unlike the pacifist who refuses to pay taxes, but the moral question to be answered is the same. Is it right to opt out in order to keep my own conscience clear? Paradoxically, this *might* be merely a selfish action, since abortion procedures (like expenditure on armaments) will continue with the rest of one's fellow nurses still involved. We would respect a nurse whose conscience prevented her from taking part in abortions, yet we might equally admire the one who, despite the moral conflict entailed, chose to carry on, realising that opting out put a greater burden on colleagues. We recognise that people may sometimes feel obliged to remain involved in a morally ambiguous situation in order to share the difficulties with their fellow human beings rather than simply choosing the action which keeps their own moral principles intact.

Already it is plain that conscience-following is a much

more complicated affair than Butler seemed to realise. If one might feel an obligation to *disregard* one's conscience, then the implication is that to obey conscience is not necessarily the only way of acting rightly. Another example may bring this point home more clearly:

This episode happened while I was on night duty in an intensive care ward. One of the patients, a boy aged seven years, was being kept alive on a ventilator. In addition he had a pace-maker inserted into his heart. In a case of this kind it is sometimes difficult to determine when a patient actually dies. At one point it appeared that this had in fact happened. The doctor was informed and on coming to see the boy felt uncertain whether the patient was dead. In the end he decided that he was. A nurse was then asked to turn off the machines, even though the cardiometer showed some signs of the heart still functioning. The doctor explained to the nurse that the boy most likely had brain damage due to the length of time that he had been starved of a supply of oxygenated blood to the brain cells. Therefore (the doctor argued), even if the patient weren't dead, it would be better if he died now rather than survive to be a 'hopeless case'. Despite these arguments the nurse felt that her conscience would not allow her to obey the doctor's instructions, and the doctor switched off the machines himself.

This example illustrates the purely *personal* reference of the guidance of conscience. Here is a situation in which a nurse feels that the same action is permissible for the doctor but not permissible for her. (If this had *not* been so, she would surely have been obliged to intervene in what she must regard as murder.) In effect what the nurse is saying to the doctor is: 'I see that the arguments you give are sufficient for you to feel that you are doing the right thing by switching off the machine. I don't doubt that you are acting according to your conscience, but my conscience tells me differently.' Yet this seems a very odd state of affairs! Apart from the question of whether the doctor really ought to have tried to delegate so important an action to nursing staff, surely the action is either morally right or morally wrong irrespective of who does it.

Thus we are once more seeing a situation in which saying 'My conscience tells me not to do this' is not necessarily saying the same as 'This is absolutely wrong'. It seems that conscience is a powerful force in controlling the actions of most individuals—so powerful that we would always hesitate to ask anyone to violate it. But although powerful, it may not always be right. (*Butler* said the opposite: although right, not always powerful.) After all, if everyone's conscience always gave totally correct statements of the right actions in situations, no two consciences would ever differ. Yet, unless we suppose that everyone with different views from our own is either totally ignorant or completely unscrupulous, we know that there can be many genuine disagreements of conscience. Thus the guidance of my conscience may be right for me, but not right for somebody else.

We are tempted to conclude, from the discussion so far, that conscience has more to do with the psychological make-up of the individual than it has with the morality of actions. Faced with the evidence of the variability of conscience from person to person, it seems reasonable to suppose that, far from being an infallible guide to right and wrong, it is merely an aspect of the individual's character which has been determined by his genetic predispositions, the culture in which he has been reared and the nature of his childhood experiences. The view that conscience is culturally and psychologically conditioned has gained popularity in contemporary thought, largely as a result of the very thorough analysis of the origin of guilt in neurotic illness carried out by Sigmund Freud and other members of the psychoanalytic school of psychology. We shall therefore take our analysis of conscience a step further by examining this way of understanding it.

## Conscience and Superego

Within the confines of this chapter, drastic condensation has to be made of a mass of material on the psychological origins of conscience. The psychoanalytic theory is by no means the only current psychological analysis of conscience, and within psychoanalysis itself there is a wide range of schools of thought. All that we can hope to do is to look briefly at the main points of Freud's theory of conscience. This will serve us as an example of the type of psychological explanation that can be offered.

**Sigmund Freud** (1856–1939) formulated his psychological theories as a result of clinical psychiatric practice. It was his life-long interest in patients who showed psychoneurotic symptoms, such as hysterical paralysis of a limb, phobic reactions to enclosed spaces, or obsessive thoughts and compulsive behaviour patterns, which led him to try to conceptualise the different forces at work in both the neurotic and the 'normal' personality. Early in his career Freud discovered that if patients could be allowed to talk about experiences which upset them, an emotional release (catharsis) occurred which resulted in the alleviation of symptoms. This therapeutic technique Freud named *abreaction* and, in association with Breuer, he developed ways of bringing about abreactions, through the use of hypnosis. However, hypnotic methods, although revealing to the psychiatrist, brought no insight to the patient into the origins of his disturbance, yet insight of this kind seemed necessary for permanent cure. Freud, therefore, adopted new techniques. These were *free association* and *dream* *analysis* and they became the basic tools of the new therapeutic method he was to name *psychoanalysis*. In free association the patient, reclining in a relaxed position, was encouraged to verbalise thoughts and feelings as they came into his mind, without any attempt to organise or control them. In dream analysis the patient was encouraged to remember and record his dreams so that, with the aid of the psychoanalyst, he could explore their significance. Both methods were designed to by-pass the patient's moral editing and controlling of upsetting aspects of his experiences without blotting out awareness through a hypnotic trance. The elaborating and refining of these methods of therapy and the formulation and reformulation of psychoanalytic theory based on the use of these methods resulted in the foundation of a whole new school of psychology, which by the time of Freud's death in 1939 already had several major orthodox theorists as well as numerous heretics and revisionists (Brown, 1961).

It is important to remember the therapeutic concern behind the development of psychoanalysis when one is trying to understand any aspect of its theoretical concepts. This is perhaps especially true of the psychoanalytic account of conscience, which finds its origins in the attempt to understand the pervasiveness of guilt feelings in psychiatric disorders. In his early psychoanalytic work Freud was struck by the powerful censoring forces in the human personality which seemed to act as a kind of barrier between the patient's conscious awareness and the more sensitive areas of his experience. Attempts to explore these areas resulted in either the patient taking all sorts of evasive action (resistance) or an apparent total inability to recall experiences (repression). Freud, therefore postulated the existence of a kind of 'mental censor' which keeps large areas of our personality out of consciousness, because acknowledgment of their existence would cause unbearable anxiety. He found, through the use of free association and dream analysis, that this material was most frequently of a primitive sexual and aggressive nature and that it found its origin in patients' early childhood experiences.

The full psychoanalytic account of conscience can be seen as an explanation of how and why this censor operates with such destructive force in the creation of neurotic illness. The later theoretical formulations adopted a new terminology: the conscious and rational aspect of the personality was named the *Ego*; the hidden motivational forces were named the *Id*; the judging and censoring aspect was named the *Superego*. The Id is the most primitive region of the personality. It is characterised by a blind seeking after release of bodily tensions. The new born infant is 'all Id', knowing only the pressing needs for sustenance and security. The Ego and the Superego gradually develop as a result of the child's increased perceptual, locomotor and conceptual skills, which bring him into contact and conflict with the world outside his own immediate desires. Both Ego and Superego attempt to impose controls on the Id, the Ego according to the restrictions demanded by adaptation to the environment, the Superego according to ideals and prohibitions conveyed to the child by the parents.

In the elaboration of the concept of the Superego, which takes the place of the earlier 'mental censor' concept, we have Freud's explanation of the feelings of obligation and of guilt by which adult behaviour is regulated. The Superego consists of two parts: the 'ego ideal' which puts forward positive values for the individual to aspire to and the 'conscience' which prohibits and controls the instinctual drives of the personality. The conscience results primarily from parental control of the child through the stages of weaning, toilet training and early sexual stimulation associated with masturbation. The development reaches a crisis around the age of 5 years, when the child, in order to solve the conflict of feelings to which he is exposed, develops *internalised* control of feelings and actions. Rather than seeing the parent as an outside authority, he incorporates the parental figure into his own personality structure. When this occurs the development of the Superego is virtually completed. The child now has within himself a figure of moral authority. What the character of this 'internal parent' will be is entirely dependent upon the quality of the relationship between child and parents up to this stage. If the child has felt unloved and has been made to feel ashamed of his sexual and aggressive drives, then his Superego will be harsh, condemning and relentless in its demands. As a result neurotic symptoms of some kind are likely to develop (for case studies of the destructiveness of the Superego *see* Menninger, 1938). On the other hand a child who has experienced control in the context of positive experiences of being loved and valued is more likely to see in the parent an *ideal* with which he wishes to be identified, and his Superego may be more in harmony with the other aspects of his personality. It should be added, however, that in Freud's view, (though not in that of all his followers), the force of the sexual and aggressive drives was such that *any* imposition of social controls upon them was bound to provoke conflict and unhappiness. In his later works, especially, Freud saw anxiety and frustration as the inevitable price we have to pay for civilisation. (In an often quoted passage he remarked wryly that perhaps all that psychoanalysis can do is to transform neurotic misery into the everyday unhappiness which is the usual lot of mankind.)

We can see that in Freudian theory the foundations of the adult conscience have been laid long before childhood is over. Subsequent experience may modify and add to the childhood prohibitions and ideals, but the *motive force* of conscience is long antecedent to adult debates about the morality of actions.

Before discussing the implications of Freud's analysis of conscience for ethical theory, we may refer to some important additions which have been made to it by subsequent Freudian theorists through the exploration of *cultural variations* in child rearing patterns. Freud sometimes seemed to write as though the childhood of all mankind were set in a nineteenth-century Viennese middle class family! Obviously parents do not impose patterns of behaviour on their children in a cultural vacuum. They act as mediators of the expectations of their own particular society and historical epoch. Such influences have been extensively traced by the psychoanalyst Erik Erikson in his studies of childhood in different cultures (Erikson, 1965). Erikson has shown what striking contrasts there are between the images of ideal adult behaviour conveyed to, for example, Hopi Indian children and children of white American parents. Thus a further variable is added to the development of conscience. Not only is it affected by the particularities of family emotional interactions, it is equally coloured by images of admirable and unacceptable behaviour transmitted by the literature, religion and folklore of different cultures.

We can now summarise the psychoanalytic account of the origins of conscience: Although in adult life we may suppose that decisions reached on the basis of conscience are the result of conscious and rational deliberation, there are in fact determinants to our choices which derive from early experiences of which we are no longer aware. The guilt which we feel when we go against our conscience, the force with which it commends some actions and prohibits others, relates to the intensity of the relationship between us and our parents at a time when we were heavily dependent on them. The 'voice of conscience' is therefore really basically the parental voice, and the guidance which it gives derives from the values which they, under the influence of the culture of which they were members, transmitted to us.

## Is Conscience Purely Relative?

It would seem at first sight that this kind of psychological analysis completely undermines the usefulness of conscience as an objective guide to moral behaviour. If the operation of conscience depends upon all sorts of accidental factors like the kind of childhood a person has and the characteristics of the culture in which he is reared, then what conscience commands is entirely relative to all sorts of factors which have nothing to do with the rightness or wrongness of the actions being considered.

Yet this conclusion can be too quickly reached. We need to ask what precisely is the nature of the explanation being offered by psychoanalytic theory. The fundamental point to be remembered is that the psychoanalyst is concerned with the emotional effect of conscience rather than with the content of what it is commanding. Psychoanalysis focuses on *pathological* guilt, that is to say, guilt which has a disintegrative effect on the personality. What a person's conscience actually tells him is of relevance only so far as it helps the therapist to understand the sources of psychological conflict. For example, a person may feel an overwhelming sense of guilt about some incident of infidelity or dishonesty in his past life. The task of the therapist is not to pass a value judgment on the rightness or wrongness of the action, but to help the patient to come to terms with his guilt by re-experiencing the emotional relationships which give it such a crippling force. Psychoanalysis is a theoretical structure aimed at assisting therapy. It does not try to provide a test for moral values.

Nevertheless, even if psychoanalysis does not intend to explain away the authority of conscience, the evidence it produces for the predeterminants of conscience-following behaviour may lead one to feel that all has in fact been explained. Whether we take this view or not depends in the long run on our answer to a rather fundamental philosophical puzzle which will tend to re-appear at intervals in our study of ethical theories. This puzzle is concerned with whether tracing the antecedents of an individual's action amounts to a complete explanation of why he took that particular action (*see* Chapter Five for a discussion of this question). In the case of conscience, we have to decide whether there is such a thing as the *independent conscience*, which although greatly *influenced* by upbringing and culture, has also independence from these influences and is capable of conscious and reasoned choice of moral principles. If there can be a conscience of this type—we might call it a 'mature' conscience—then it can be argued that all human beings, whatever their cultural backgrounds and psychological make-up, are capable of developing sensitivity to fundamental human values. Disagreements over questions of conscience would be explained by the inability of some people to exercise *mature* judgment over their own background and culture.

The question of whether there can be a basic human conscience is far from being one of merely theoretical interest. Underlying it are fundamental issues to do with the possibility of a truly international system of law which does not depend on the rights or customary principles of separate states. A document like the United Nations *Statement on Human Rights* presupposes that such a trans-cultural set of values is possible, as do debates over the morality of war or of racial segregation. However, it seems unlikely that there is any way of *proving* the existence of such an entity as the basic human conscience. One might use as evidence the emergence of certain basic principles of morality across all the major moral and religious codes. But such arguments are not at all logically conclusive, since it can be asserted that the similarities are due to the fact that human beings, for all their diversities of culture, are subjected to enough similar social pressures to bring about the similarities in moral codes. Thus all we can say for the present is that, despite the tracing by psychological theory of the childhood antecedents of conscience, it is still *possible* to assert the independence of the adult conscience.

By way of illustration of the above discussion we can look at another clinical case:

A young man, who had had a strict religious upbringing, had been referred to a psychiatric hospital from a venereal disease clinic. The clinic staff had found it impossible to convince him that he did not have syphilis, following a recent illicit sexual experience. Even after a considerable time in hospital, he remained unshaken in his delusion. It was suggested by one psychiatrist that it was important that the patient should be convinced that it was not wrong to have sex outside marriage. A male nurse then attempted to change his ideas, but without success. But even if he had succeeded, was it right to try to undermine what the patient had been taught by his parents and his religion?

A surprising aspect of this example is the inept and un-professional way in which the patient seems to have been handled. Attempts to argue patients out of delusional beliefs would hardly be characteristic of most modern psychiatric practice. Apart from this, however, the example illustrates confusion between the rightness or wrongness of the principles held by conscience and pathological effects of conscience in psychiatric disorder. The view that 'sex outside marriage is wrong' would not be regarded in our culture as obviously delusional. It may or may not be correct, but certainly it is possible to argue rationally about it. The problem for the patient was the intensity of the guilt which transgressing such a principle created, and this in turn seems to have been related to the strict parental authority still haunting the patient's conscience. Had the male nurse succeeded in his ambitious project and convinced the patient, the hospital would most likely have then had to deal with someone excessively guilty about *not* having sex outside marriage! The aim of psychiatric intervention in a situation like this is not to instil any particular set of moral values into the patient, but to free him from the irrational control of infantile aspects of his personality so that he can adopt whatever set of moral principles *he chooses*. Thus we return to the same point: Despite all that can be said about the potentially destructive aspects of conscience and about its relativity to the personal history of an individual, there remains the important possibility that *maturity and independence of moral choice* can be attained and that these in the long run will provide the surest guide to right action.

## The Individual and his Decisions

It would seem, then, that the common sense notion of conscience cannot easily be dispensed with in discussing moral dilemmas. Yet we should not suppose that it will necessarily be of much help to us in finding a way through the moral problems of clinical practice. We have argued, against attempts to explain away conscience, that individuals may attain maturity and independence in their decisions. However, such statements, however correct they may be, do not take us very far in settling disagreements over matters of morality. For, in cases of disagreement who is to say which person's conscience is the mature one? In the debate over the Abortion Act, for example, do we say that the Roman Catholic opponents of abortion have unemancipated consciences? Or is it that those who fear the unhappiness of the unwanted baby have suffered deprivation in their own childhood? In the debate over voluntary euthanasia is it the sign of an educated conscience to support or to oppose the right of a patient to request his own death? Clearly terms like 'mature', 'emancipated' or 'educated' very quickly degenerate in discussions of this kind into ways of asserting that your point of view is the right one.

How can we know when a person's conscience can be trusted? There appear to be only two answers to this question: One is to assert that there is no appeal beyond the individual's decision to act in one way or another. Each person must simply do what is *right for him*, even if it contradicts what is right for other individuals. In such a view all we can hope for in a society is the maximum toleration of individual difference. The other way out of the difficulty is to provide a way of discrimination between the immature and the mature conscience in terms of the use of reasoned argument. The person with a mature conscience would be able to back up his principles with reasoned arguments, whilst the person whose conscience was conditioned by his background could only continue to assert irrationally that such and such an action is right, although he can give no reason for saying it is.

The second kind of answer in fact takes us *beyond* conscience theory, since it judges between consciences according to whether their dictates can be supported by arguments. Such an appeal to reasoned argument is an acknowledgment that the individual's conscience is not the final test of rightness. We shall, therefore, leave to later chapters the discussion of what the arguments backing up conscience might be, and concentrate for the remainder of this chapter on the first alternative: that of the isolated individual making decisions valid for him and him alone.

The idea that in moral dilemmas all we are left with ultimately is the individual's personal decision has found many forms in the history of ethics. At times it has been the basis of an argument denying the possibility of genuine moral action and dismissing all attempts to formulate theories of ethics as mere wishful thinking. (Anyone who tries to make sense of the diversity of ethical theories would do well to keep this possibility in mind, although the view that all ethical theorising is futile is perhaps only honestly reached after thorough attempts to understand the whole range of theories that have been put forward.) Not all writers who stress the individual character of moral choice, however, do so in order to back up a totally sceptical view of ethics. During the last hundred years a powerful form of individualistic approach has grown up under the name of Existentialism, which is of particular relevance to our concern with moral dilemmas. The existentialist philosophers take the concerns of moral philosophy entirely seriously, seeing in the agonies of moral dilemmas a critical point of illumination for understanding the genuinely human.

Existentialism is not correctly seen as a *school* of philosophy (where this term is understood to mean an accepted body of theory elaborated by a number of theorists), but rather as a *way of doing* philosophy, with which the names of several philosophers are loosely associated, some of whom would recognise the title others of whom would not. The approach to existentialist philosophy is characterised by a stress on the openness to the future of human existence. Human beings are set apart from the world in which they are set by the *possibilities of choice* constantly before them. The existentialist sees the individual not as someone whose life is predetermined in some external way, but as a person who may chose what he will become. This emphasis is summed up in a slogan often used to epitomise the existentialist position: Existence precedes Essence.

The nineteenth-century Danish philosopher-theologian **Soren Kierkegaard** (1813–55) is usually identified as the 'father' of existentialism. His writings represented a violent protest against the system-building of the philosophers and theologians of his age. In all Kierkegaard's works there is a passionate defence of subjectivity, of the individual in the moment of decision as the only point of importance in beginning the search for truth. In his own time Kierkegaard was seen largely as an eccentric and his work sank into obscurity until the early part of the twentieth century, when several versions of existentialist thought began to be developed, both in philosophy and in theology.

It would be out of harmony with the whole atmosphere of existentialism to try to summarise some common set of ideas held by the many different writers now associated with this approach. All that it is possible to do is to select one writer and attempt to convey some of his basic assertions. From the point of view of the development of ethical theory the work of the French philosopher, novelist and playwright **Jean-Paul Sartre** (1905– ) is the most easily dealt with. Sartre's thought pivots on two aspects of human existence—the terrifying freedom which man has to make choices in a life in which there are no guaranteed right and wrong choices; and man's tendency to escape from so unnerving a freedom by seeking refuge in some general explanation of what is really a meaningless universe. Sartre uses a particular set of terms to characterise these different aspects. His denial of any ultimate meaning in (or explanation for) the world and human life he conveys by the use of the word 'absurd'. The man who faces reality without self-deception, faces up to its absurdity: To see this absurdity of existence coupled with man's freedom to choose is to experience both 'nausea' and 'anguish'. There is no sense in things yet one *must* choose. In such a situation one feels a dizziness, a nausea and any decision taken must bring a feeling of 'anguish', for one knows one will never find an ultimate justification for it. Not surprisingly human beings find such awareness of their futility hard to tolerate and therefore, they frequently resort to 'bad faith' (*mauvaise foi*), deluding themselves with some dogmatism, whether religious or materialistic. For authentic human existence, however, there is no escape from the harshness of the choices which the individual must make for himself and for which he, and he alone, must take responsibility.

An example used by Sartre himself may serve to convey the essence of his philosophy. It is given by him as an illustration of the fact that the individual is entirely alone, abandoned in his decisions:

As an example by which you may the better understand this state of abandonment, I will refer to the case of a pupil of mine, who sought me out in the following circumstances. His father was quarrelling with his mother and was also inclined to be a 'collaborator'; his elder brother had been killed in the German offensive of 1940 and this young man, with a sentiment somewhat primitive but generous, burned to avenge him.

His mother was living alone with him, deeply afflicted by the semi-treason of his father and by the death of her eldest son, and her one consolation was in this young man. But he, at this moment, had the choice between going to England to join the Free French Forces or of staying near his mother and helping her to live. He fully realised that this woman lived only for him and that his disappearance—or perhaps his death —would plunge her into despair. He also realised that, concretely and in fact, every action he performed on his mother's behalf would be sure of effect in the sense of aiding her to live, whereas anything he did in order to go and fight would be an ambiguous action which might vanish like water into sand and serve no purpose. . . . Consequently, he found himself confronted by two very different modes of action; the one concrete immediate but directed towards only one individual; and the other an action addressed to an end infinitely greater, a national collectivity, but for that very reason ambiguous—and it might be frustrated on the way. At the same time he was hesitating between two kinds of morality; on the one side the morality of sympathy of personal devotion and, on the other side, a morality of wider scope but of more debatable validity. He had to choose between those two. What could help him to choose? Could the Christian doctrine? No. Christian doctrine says: Act with charity, love your neighbour, deny yourself for others, choose the way which is hardest, and so forth. But which is the harder road? To whom does one owe the more brotherly love, the patriot or the mother? Which is the more useful aim, the general one of fighting in and for the whole community, or the precise aim of helping one particular person to live? Who can give an answer to that a priori? No one. (Sartre, 1948, p. 35.)

Little more can be said in a general way about existentialist ethics. It will be evident that it begins and ends with the individual and his decisions and that most of its further exposition is concerned with identifying attempts to find false ways out of the pain of decision-making. Behind such a view there lies an extensive discussion of the nature of human thought and action. Indeed the main bulk of existentialist writing is concerned with wider philosophical questions about the different manifestations of 'being' in human and non-human existence, rather than with the particular questions which occupy the attention of ethical theorists. Thus we are not really, as may have been obvious even in the brief glimpse we have had of Sartre, dealing with an elaborate ethical theory, but rather with a way of regarding moral choice.

It may also become clear that an essential component of a point of view like Sartre's is the fundamental assumption that there is no ultimate meaning in life. Perhaps because of the utter isolation of the individual in existentialist thought, the assertion or denial of religious faith is a critical question for many of its proponents. Thus for Sartre the assertion of Absurdity is all important. Other existentialists, such as Kierkegaard or Tillich, have made religious affirmations the foundation of their philosophy, but the difference between the religious and non-religious existentialists is perhaps not really great so far as their view of moral choice is concerned. For both the question of *ultimate meaning* is central, since, in order to take on the full responsibility of personal decision the individual must settle that question one way or another. The man of total faith and the man of total unfaith are perhaps not so very different in the resoluteness of their moral choices. Each has made his mind up about the significance of his life within the whole context of human existence.

## Summary: The Limits of Conscience Theory

We now seem to have followed the 'plain man's' feeling that his conscience knows best just about as far as it will take us. In a nutshell we might say that such a view seems sensible enough until we meet two plain men who disagree. Then we have to think more carefully about what we mean by conscience. Do some consciences know better than others? This question becomes more acute when we realise how many powerful influences are at work moulding a wide variety of consciences. In order to retain its usefulness it seems either that conscience must be subject to some sort of test which will sort out the reliable consciences from the unreliable ones, or that we have to accept utter individuality of moral viewpoint as an inevitable aspect of the human situation.

This second possibility, in the form of the existentialist account of moral decision, has now been outlined. It represents a limit in ethical theory at which it is perfectly possible to come to rest. No-one would claim for it the qualities of a comfortable or convenient resting place, but then these are hardly to be expected from the high-minded pursuit of morality! In addition its individuality presents serious problems for social organisation, since no-one has the right to say of another decision—provided that it was taken in good faith—that it is morally culpable. In a situation where the majority of people were existentialist in outlook, matters of policy and day-to-day decision in the administration of any large organisation could become exceedingly complex not to say unpredictable. This means that existentialism is a difficult philosophy to use as a base from which to understand the kind of dilemmas facing doctors and nurses, since it seems that the whole philosophy of the medical endeavour rests on the assumption that there *can* be a set of shared values about health, happiness and the quality of human life, even if these values are often difficult to articulate clearly. Much emphasis certainly is placed on the carrying of responsibility for individual decision within medical practice and for this reason the existentialist stress on the crucial nature of choice is highly relevant to the doctor faced with a tricky clinical situation. But the search for a *consensus* in moral values is as relevant an aspect of the contemporary scene as the lone clinician and his agonised decision. The questions facing medicine at the present time are so closely tied with questions of social policy and economic priorities that they demand collective rather than individual decisions both within the health professions and within the whole society whose health priorities must be decided. To such problems existentialism seems to say little except that it is futile to seek for general solutions.

Of course, the points we have been making in criticism of an overstress on individualism in ethics in no sense prove existentialism to be wrong. Sartre's calm acceptance of absurdity may, for all we know, be the only sanity possible. Such criticisms merely suggest that we might well examine some alternative solutions, before accepting that no appeal beyond conscience is possible. Such solutions are offered by theories which look for so-called 'objective' measures of right and wrong, that is to say, measures which go outside the individual apprehension of moral values. In the chapters which follow we shall explore several theories of this type.

## REFERENCES

Brown, J. A. C. (1961). *Freud and the Post-Freudians.* London: Penguin.

Butler, J. (1970). *Fifteen Sermons.* Ed. Roberts, T. A. (First published 1726.) London: S.P.C.K.

Erikson, E. H. (1965). *Childhood and Society.* London: Penguin.

Menninger, K. A. (1938). *Man Against Himself*. New York: Harcourt, Brace and World.

Sartre, J.-P. (1948) *Existentialism and Humanism*. London: Methuen.

Wright, D. (1971). *The Psychology of Moral Behaviour*. London: Penguin.

# CHAPTER THREE

# The Common Good

The birth of a spina bifida baby provokes difficult moral choices. Treatment of such cases varies according to the views of the receiving surgeon. In one hospital it is the policy of surgeon A to operate immediately in order to minimise the risk of the lesion becoming infected. Surgeon B will wait two or three days in order to assess the baby's chance of survival and discuss the prognosis with the father. On what basis should the discussion to intervene surgically be made? Should it be decided according to the ethics of the surgeon, the attitude of the parents or the willingness of our society to provide proper facilities for the severely handicapped? How are we to judge what is best for the child?

The staffing of hospital departments poses the problems of where to give priority in numbers of trained staff and total numbers of staff. Two extremes of this problem in a psychiatric hospital are the child psychiatry unit and the geriatric wards. The children require almost individual attention and so do the old people because of their frailty and the risk of accidents. When there is less than the ideal number of staff how should the allocations be made? Children still have life ahead of them. Perhaps the old should have the bare minimum for the sake of the possible benefit to the young. Or should the children have a little less care in order to give more comfort to the older people who have given to others for years?

The questions posed by these examples illustrate the kind of debate over priorities in medicine which demands the establishment of a shared basis for decision-making in the moral choices facing doctors, nurses and the societies of which they are members. Whatever the decisions taken about allocation of resources to the elderly, to the severely handicapped or to patients whose treatment requires heavy expenditure, it does not seem appropriate that they should depend solely on the personal moral views of individuals. Some general moral guide-lines need to be found which will assist the decisions of individuals.

It appears at first glance that such a guide-line should be found in the notion of *the common good*. Decisions about priorities would be taken in the light of the likely consequences for all those directly and indirectly involved, the aim being to bring as much all round benefit as possible to the majority without causing undue suffering to any minorities. Thus *avoiding pain and maximising happiness for the greatest number of people* becomes the formula for determining right decisions in any situation or moral dilemma. The exposition and criticism of this point of view, which is known as the Greatest Happiness Theory or Utilitarianism ('greatest usefulness') will occupy us for the whole of this chapter. The general principle of right and wrong which it offers is clearly intimately connected to the philosophy of the practice of medicine, which takes as its basis the alleviation of suffering and the promotion of health amongst humanity as a whole. The question we must answer is whether its concept of 'the common good' is adequate to the task of determining what we mean by morally right and wrong actions in the medical endeavour

## Happiness and Morality

The contention that happiness and morality are intimately connected has been put forward in many forms throughout the history of ethical theorising. The general description for theories which make such a link-up is 'hedonistic', a term which derives from the Greek word *hedone* meaning 'pleasure'. One of the most widely known (and misunderstood) versions of Hedonism is that of the Greek philosopher **Epicurus** (341–270 B.C.), who asserted that man ought to devote his life to the cultivation of his own long-term happiness. Epicurus was far from advocating the kind of living for the pleasures of the moment with which the description 'Epicurean' is often wrongly associated. Rather, he was putting forward the *achievement of a state of happiness* as an ultimate value in morality. To achieve this the individual might require much self-discipline and was advised to pursue the pleasures of the mind in preference to those of the body.

Hedonistic theories can be divided into two main types: those which, like Epicureanism, assert that man *ought* to seek happiness, are known as *ethical* hedonistic theories: those which assert more simply that all men *are in fact* motivated only by the drive for happiness are known as *psychological* hedonistic theories. Both ethical and psychological hedonism can take either (a) an individualistic form; or (b) a universalistic form, by asserting either (a) that men ought to or do in fact seek *their own happiness* only; or (b) that men ought to or do in fact seek *the happiness of everyone*.

Out of this wide range of possible theories we are selecting only one: the universalistic ethical type, which states that the basis for moral action *ought* to be the achievement of happiness for everyone, even though many individuals may not in fact use this as a basis. Because of its similarity to the ideals of a health service, the 'universal happiness' form seems the obvious place to start our assessment of hedonism. In a later chapter (Chapter Five) we shall return to the psychological form of hedonism, which states that all human action is motivated by the drive for pleasure.

The English philosopher and political theorist **John Stuart Mill** (1806–73) provides us with the most comprehensive (although not the most consistent) form of universalistic ethical hedonism. Mill was heavily involved in the movements towards social and political reform of his time. He served for a period as a Member of Parliament, but his main influence was exerted by his political and ethical writings, especially his essays, *On Liberty* and *Utilitarianism*. Mill found his inspiration in the political fervour of his father James Mill and particularly in the ethical theory propounded by James Mill's friend and fellow campaigner, Jeremy Bentham. Bentham stated quite baldly that morality consisted in obtaining *the maximum amount of happiness for the greatest number of people*. Moreover, Bentham declared, it should be perfectly possible to work out a formula for calculating the amount of happiness obtained from any action. In the calculation each person should count as one and no-one as more than one and the total *quantity* of happiness accruing was all that mattered. 'Quantity of pleasure being equal' Bentham wrote, 'pushpin is as good as poetry.' (Pushpin was a game of chance—in modern terms: 'bingo is as good as poetry'.)

Let us look in a preliminary way at how this theory, based on the calculation of maximum happiness, would deal with the examples at the beginning of this chapter. It is difficult to see what possible argument there could be for the preserving of the life of the severely handicapped child on Bentham's philosophy. The child himself must count only as one and against him must be weighed the cost in effort and expense which will have to be met to support him, a cost which can never be repaid by any contribution to society by the child. Moreover, even the consideration of the pleasures possibly accruing to those most intimately involved—the parent, the medical staff, and the child himself—by saving the life of the patient, might easily be counterbalanced by the subsequent uncertainty of his condition and the work, worry and pain which this might entail. Thus the greatest happiness of the the greatest number would best be served by diverting the money and medical expertise elsewhere and not attempting any form of surgical intervention. In the case of the allocation of staff to different hospital wards, a Benthamite would have to estimate whether greater general happiness will accrue by favouring the elderly or favouring the young. It would appear that, on a purely quantitative basis, investment of resources must be in the young, since whatever the amount of happiness created by careful nursing of geriatric patients it will in the nature of things be of a shorter duration. Rehabilitation of emotionally disturbed children, on the other hand, will have much more long-term effects on the happiness of the majority.

We are not concerned at the moment with discussing whether the conclusions reached by these applications of Bentham's theory are right or wrong. This will require a much more extensive discussion. What we should observe at this stage is that this kind of 'maximum happiness' approach seems to dismiss very lightly other considerations to do with respect for life and care of individuals for their own sakes, which are normally of great importance in questions of medical morality. Bentham's theory, although it was the basis for much humanitarian reform, seems a crude and inhuman approach in these applications of it. The refinement of its rough and ready standard of morality brings us to the writings of John Stuart Mill.

Mill regarded Bentham's philosophy as the only possible basis for a rational analysis of morality, but he attempted to moderate its wilder statements by introducing more subtlety into the concept of maximum happiness. His basic definition of the 'Greatest Happiness Principle' sounds similar to Bentham's:

'... actions are right in proportion as they tend to promote happiness, wrong as they tend to produce the reverse of happiness. By happiness is intended pleasure and the absence of pain; by unhappiness, pain and the privation of pleasure.' (*Utilitarianism*, p. 9.)

This definition, however, was then modified in a number of ways which quite changed the character of the theory. Firstly, Mill did not agree with Bentham's equation of 'Pushpin and poetry', but wished to include a difference in *quality* of pleasure as well as a difference in quantity. Like Epicurus, Mill believed that the pleasures of the mind were of a different order from the pleasures of the body, even though it might be easier to satisfy the latter. 'It is better' he wrote in *Utilitarianism*, 'to be a human being dissatisfied than a pig satisfied; better to be Socrates dissatisfied than a fool satisfied'. Thus in estimating what was right in any situation we would have to take into account the *kind* as well as the amount of happiness likely to result from alternative courses of action. But how were such estimations of quality to be made? Here Mill appealed to the concept of the *competent judge*. Only the person who has known both 'higher' and 'lower' pleasures is competent to judge between them. Thus Socrates is a better judge of happiness than a fool. (This modification of the quantitative version of hedonism bristles with difficulties, not the least of which is the problem of finding competent judges of happiness—philosophers may be the last people to look to for such a skill! But we shall leave discussion of these problems aside for the present and examine the other adaptations of the greatest happiness principle which Mill introduced.)

Mill's second modification was the admission that, although in *theory* the greatest happiness principle was the only ultimate test of rightness, in practice it was by no means easy to use it in the solution of dilemmas. He did not share Bentham's happy confidence in the possibility of a 'felicific calculus'—a formula whereby, by taking into account such factors as intensity, duration and fruitfulness of other pleasures, the pleasurable or painful consequences of any action could be worked out. Because he was aware of the subtleties in the human perception of happiness, Mill realised that many of the problems of personal and social morality facing his contemporaries required a complex balancing of one set of advantages against another. Yet Mill felt that at any rate no better test of rightness was likely to be found than that of greatest happiness. Even if difficult to apply, such a test was at least 'tangible and intelligible'. All men, he argued, know what it is to suffer pain and experience pleasure. Even although their estimations of the happy life may vary, at least they agree on seeing happiness as a goal to be striven for both for themselves and for their fellow men.

The third modification of general happiness theory which Mill introduced is so drastic that it leads us to call his viewpoint a *greatest benefit* (or 'utilitarian') theory rather than a pure example of a *greatest happiness* (or 'hedonistic') theory. Happiness, Mill argued, is not a simple concept referring one kind of experience. Rather it denotes the achievement of a number of beneficial experiences such as the awareness of beauty, the exercise of virtue or the experience of health, which are valued for themselves. Here is how Mill himself puts it in Chapter Four of *Utilitarianism*:

'The ingredients of happiness are very various, and each

of them is desirable in itself, and not merely when considered as swelling an aggregate. The principle of utility does not mean that any given pleasure, as music, for instance, or any given exemption from pain, as for example health, are to be looked upon as means to a collective something called happiness and to be desired on that account. They are desired and desirable in and for themselves; besides being a means, they are part of an end.'

We see clearly from this quotation that Mill is using the word 'happiness' to refer to all those things which he sees as of ultimate value in human life. Thus his theory is really a 'common good' or 'benefit of the majority' theory. To act rightly is to work towards the distributing as widely as possible of those human experiences (such as freedom, health, awareness of beauty and of truth), which bring the highest fulfilment to individual lives. We have come a long way from the simple notion that acting rightly means maximising happiness. Mill's sensitive awareness of the complexity of human experience made him incapable of defending consistently a philosophy based on pleasure alone. This is nowhere more evident than in his powerful defence of freedom of the individual in the essay *On Liberty*, which passionately opposes the imposition of conformity for the sake of social benefit:

'The worth of a State, in the long run, is the worth of the individuals composing it; ... a State which dwarfs its men in order that they may be more docile instruments in its hands even for beneficial purposes—will find that with small men no great thing can be accomplished.'

## Utilitarianism and the Welfare State

It would be difficult to overstate the influence of utilitarian philosophy on the social and political changes which began in nineteenth-century Britain and have continued up to the present time. Whatever its crudities or inconsistencies, it was the philosophy of Bentham and Mill which lay behind reforms in conditions of employment, in the prison system, in public health provision, in parliamentary representation and in the status of women. One social historian sums up the influence of utilitarianism as follows: '... Bentham founded a school of thought which, developing and changing in the hands of his disciples as the century progressed, provided a dynamic force of legal, social, political and economic reform, and a touchstone for all governmental policies' (Thomson, 1950, p. 30). Particularly relevant to the concerns of this book is the link between utilitarianism and the development of public provision of health services in Britain, which culminated in the formation of the National Health Service in 1948. We shall look briefly at this development (for a full account *see* Eckstein, 1964; Willcocks, 1967), since it provides us with a 'case study' of the interrelationship of the concept of general happiness with the concept of health.

An immediate link between utilitarianism and health measures is provided in the person of Edwin Chadwick, author of a famous survey entitled *The Report on the Sanitary Condition of the Labouring Population* and the first secretary of the Poor Law Board, which was set up in 1834 to administer the workhouse system. Chadwick was an ardent disciple of Bentham's and applied the concept of the happiness of the majority to the clamant need for sanitary conditions in the urban slums created by the Industrial Revolution. His report demonstrated that expectation of life was much lower in the urban areas and that diseases like cholera (which killed 160,000 people in Britain in 1832–33) were concentrated in the most insanitary areas of the cities. Chadwick advocated the setting up of centralised authorities to deal with paving, drainage, water supply and other essential sanitary matters. The report was published in 1842, but no government action was taken until 1848, when a second cholera epidemic was on the horizon. Then, in a belated attempt to deal with the epidemic (this one was to kill 130,000), the first national Board of Health for England and Wales was set up, with Chadwick as one of its members. The principle had been established that the community as a whole should take statutory responsibility for preventing disease amongst all its members.

The development of public health measures through the nineteenth century has been well documented elsewhere (Longmate, 1966; Flinn, 1968). Our interest, however, lies in the *kind of argument* used by Chadwick in support of his reforms. Improving sanitary conditions, he reasoned, was *good economics*, since it ensured that a disease did not threaten the labour supply for the factories and saved the state the cost of maintaining widows and orphans. 'It is an appalling fact' he wrote in his *Report*, 'that, of all who are born of the labouring classes in Manchester, more than fifty-seven per cent die before they attain five years of age, that is, before they can be engaged in factory labour'. Thus public health reforms were introduced because it was expedient for the community that the cities should be cleaned up, not because the slum dwellers had any inherent right to decent living conditions. We see in this argument the quantitative assessment of maximum happiness of Bentham's philosophy. Although of course there were in the reform movements of the time many men motivated by arguments of a quite different kind from this one, the stress on the *usefulness* of public health legislation was a very strong one. The kernel of the argument is to be found in the *Fourth Annual Report of the Poor Law Commis-*

*sioners* (1838): 'All epidemics, and all infectious diseases, are attended with charges, immediate and ultimate, on the poor rates ... The amount of burthens thus produced is frequently so great as to render it good economy on the part of the administrators of the Poor Law to incur the charges for preventing the evils where they are ascribable to physical causes'.

The transition from public health legislation in the nineteenth century to the concept of a national health service in the twentieth marks a significant shift in moral values. The Beveridge Report, a hundred years after Chadwick's report, states as one of its main assumptions that: '... a comprehensive national health service will ensure that for every citizen there is available *whatever medical treatment he requires,* in whatever form he requires it ...' (*National Health Service Act*, Section 1, my italics). The assumption now is *not* that the prevention of disease is good economy, but that every citizen has the *right* to receive whatever treatment is necessary for his health. The spirit of this approach to health legislation is captured in the following vision of a new post-war Britain, painted by Lord Woolton, then Minister of Reconstruction, in a speech delivered in 1945. He pictured a society 'that resolved to share to the full in the protection of the individual from the evils of misfortune that come from the mischance of ill-health or unemployment, and a society that was resolved to use all the powers of government and finance for the purpose of raising the standard of our common life and for our fuller enjoyment of the beauties of life and the art of living' (quoted in Ross, 1952, p. 10).

It would be easy to oversimplify and glamourise the shift from the assumptions of Chadwick to the assumptions of Beveridge and the many other figures involved in the creation of the British 'welfare state': Chroniclers of the birth of the National Health Service have shown that it was the outcome of a complex series of political negotiations (*see* especially Willcocks, 1967). But although there was much uncertainty about the details of the administrative structures introduced (and debate over this continues), the *principle* of equal distribution of medical provision according to need was accepted and practised by the medical profession long before the National Health Service Act and the philosophy of the Beveridge Report was enthusiastically endorsed across political party lines.

It is this change from the principle of the social usefulness of public hygiene to the principle of the responsibility of society for the *health of each individual* which is of interest to us, since it illustrates the problems which emerge when one moves from a Benthamite quantitative approach to the form of utilitarianism propounded by Mill, which stresses the quality of each individual life. As the National Health Service has faced up to its statutory obligation to provide 'a comprehensive health service designed to secure improvement in the physical and mental health of the people' it has become obvious that there can never be sufficient resources to meet all the health needs of every individual. The resulting dilemma is well expressed in an assessment by representatives of the medical profession of the first 10 years of the operation of the NHS:

'For the doctor the primary concern when confronted by a patient physically or mentally sick is to restore that patient to health as quickly as possible. The fact that a doctor is working in a service financed and organised by the State should not be allowed to affect this fundamental duty. On the other hand, no-one—least of all the doctor—can fail to be aware of the many legitimate and competing demands demands within the service for the money available. In theory there is no absolute ceiling on National Health Service expenditure, but in practice there will always be a limit to the amount of public money and the extent of the country's economic resources which can be devoted to this end' (Medical Services Review Committee, para. 37).

How then are priorities in expenditure to be decided? It would seem to be totally out of harmony with the legislation to adopt a Benthamite principle of benefit to the economy. Many classes of patient—the mentally subnormal or the senile, for example—have little or no contribution to make to the national productivity. The question is one which has to be answered in many different contexts ranging from the parliamentary debates over the national budget through to allocations of funds by regional hospital boards to decisions about treatment by individual clinicians. Thus the humanitarian philosophy upon which the National Health Service is based provokes in a very concrete form a set of problems to do with the equitable distribution of health resources. Is the modified greatest happiness theory of J. S. Mill able to cope with these problems? We shall attempt to answer this question by relating a series of criticisms of Mill's theory to some specific clinical situations. The first two criticisms centre round practical difficulties in the theory: how is happiness to be defined? and how can happiness be predicted?; the third criticism focuses on the fundamental issue of whether happiness can be used as a way of defining rightness.

## Defining Happiness

In the discussion so far we have been using the terms 'pleasure' and 'happiness' interchangeably, without offering a definition of either. This kind of haziness in the use of terms is one of the difficulties in a theory like Mill's. We might locate the terms 'pain', 'pleasure' and 'happiness' on a scale of increasing vagueness. The experience of *pain* is normally easily recognised and named. Although individuals seem to vary in 'pain threshold', and although the concept of 'mental pain' or 'psychological pain' can cause problems, on the whole it is possible to get broad agreement both on what constitutes pain and on the principle that it is something to be avoided unless there are good reasons for tolerating it. Pleasure is less easy to define and evaluate. Sometimes it is equated with the absence of pain, or with the experience of relief from pain, but this seems inadequate to convey the positive aspects of the experience. Further description can be offered in terms of the relief from bodily tensions of various sorts. Thus pleasure is exemplified in the relief of hunger pangs or the satisfaction of sexual needs. Yet many pleasures seem to be only vaguely related to basic bodily needs. (The pleasures of the gourmet for example are not explicable by referring to the state of his appetite only.) Very rapidly, we find that the scope of experience covered by the word 'pleasure' is extremely wide. Moreover as the range widens it seems impossible to find any common feature in the experiences except the general observation that 'people enjoy them'. (Certainly one can offer ingenious psychological hypotheses about the common features of, say reading a novel, watching a football match and scratching an itch, but the theoretical concepts offered seem to miss the essence of the actual experience of pleasure.) The question of evaluation also becomes acute as the variety of pleasure increases. People differ so much in what they find pleasurable that there is little common agreement about which experiences are to be sought after. Again, the 'pursuit of pleasure' seems less obviously good in itself than the avoidance of pain. Indeed pleasures are often divided into the innocent and the not so innocent, or the whole experience of pleasure is dismissed as irrelevant to the good life. Into this conceptual tangle, the term *happiness* is frequently introduced as a way of distinguishing between the immediate gratification of pleasurable experiences, which may or may not be morally valuable, and the long-term satisfaction of the individual in all his aspects. Thus 'happiness' is used to mean something like 'fulfilment of the whole personality'.

It is this broad conception of happiness that Mill seemed to be aiming for in his attempt to distinguish between qualities of pleasure and his admission that certain things like virtue or health were valuable in themselves and not just valued for the pleasure they bring. But although introducing the concept of happiness may do more justice to the complexity of human experience, it fails to give any clarity to the definition of right and wrong. We are left now with a concept even less clearly defined and even more open to disagreement than the concept of pleasure. For, who is to decide what fulfils human beings or what experiences are to be given the status of ingredients of happiness? As we saw earlier, Mill thought that we would appeal to the 'competent judge', who, having had experience of all kinds of pleasure, would be able to discriminate between 'higher' and 'lower' ones. We can agree certainly that we respect the judgment of people of wide experience and fine discrimination and may look to them for guidance, but we would never regard such opinion as binding and infallible. We realise that their judgment might be faulty and their long experience might in some instances limit rather than clarify their vision. What Mill failed to see was that his argument ran round in a circle: the judges we call 'competent' are those who point us toward experiences which we also would judge as higher or better—we would soon dismiss as 'incompetent' an individual who, however broad his experience, constantly opted for what we considered 'lower' pleasures. Thus we judge competence in terms of our own views of the quality of pleasure, *yet* the appeal to the competent judge was an attempt to get beyond the uncertainty of individual judgment.

The same difficulty arises with Mill's description of the ingredients of happiness. What he is saying seems a good reflection of human experience: many experiences, like the search for understanding or the appreciation of beauty, carry their own value. We do not need to justify them by saying that they result in some other experience called 'pleasure'. We *enjoy* them, of course, but that enjoyment is only one aspect of an activity which we consider worthwhile in any case. Why then does Mill need to use the word 'happiness' at all? It seems to add nothing to what he has already said, since he has now divorced it from the concept of pleasure and made it mean the same as 'those experiences which are valuable in themselves'. Just as in the case of the competent judge, we have come round in a circle: happiness was supposed to be a test of value, but now value becomes the test of 'true' happiness.

It would appear then that the definition of happiness, and its near relatives pleasure and pain, is a major problem in greater happiness theory. In fairness to Mill, it should be noted that he readily admitted that in cases of serious disagreement about right and wrong the utilitarian test of morality was not likely to provide an easy solution, although he felt convinced that at least it was better than any of the alternatives offered in other ethical theories. Yet the difficulties in the application of the concept of happiness are surely much greater than he realised. We can find clear illustrations of these difficulties if we look at decisions about medical care.

We have already seen that, in Bentham's form of the theory, many classes of patient would come very low on a list of priorities, because of the low benefit to the community as a whole of devoting disproportionate attention to them. This kind of conclusion would not be tolerated in Mill's version of the theory, in which the *quality* of happiness made available to a few would counterbalance any possible financial loss to the many. But although Mill would rule out gross neglect of the elderly and the subnormal (as would the Benthamites in practice although their *theory* might have allowed it), it is not clear how his distinction in qualities of pleasure can help to settle the more subtle questions of priority. Is there a greater quality of pleasure involved in saving the lives of a few more patients suffering from renal failure or in financing a more efficient community based geriatric service? On Mill's system, we do not regard merely the greater number of the elderly, but the quality of the experience being made available. Yet who can possibly estimate the difference in quality between the chance given to an old person to live in their own home rather than being put in an institutional setting and the opportunity to a young mother to stay with her family, although on a limited basis for a few more years? If the latter is felt to be greater in quality than the former, what then happens to the calculation when we measure the greater quality of happiness of a few against the lesser quality of happiness of many? We see that, far from simplifying the calculations, Mill's addition of the dimension of quality, renders the 'arithmetic of happiness' insoluble.

As a way out of this kind of problem in medical decision-making it is often suggested : (1) that doctors must concern themselves only with the patient for whom they have clinical responsibility at the time and must act in accordance with his best interests; and (2) that medicine does not and cannot attempt to make people happy, but only to remove the obstacles to happiness in the form of disability, malfunctioning and pain. These two important limitations on moral responsibility in medical practice do certainly simplify the matter of choice of priorities, but it would be wrong to suppose either that they are absolute or that they solve all the difficulties inherent in greatest happiness theory. The principle of responsibility to the individual patient is one to which we shall return at the end of the chapter and again later in the book, but for the moment we can observe that medical participation in the administration of the health service makes it inevitable that priorities in medicine become the concern of practitioners, even although they ought not to think in terms of priorities when confronted by the individual patient. The second point, limiting medicine to the alleviation of the distress, helps to keep the scope of medical care within manageable bounds, yet in fact the borderline between removing disability and promoting happiness is not easily drawn. This is especially true when health is broadened to include community mental health, but the following cases illustrate how, even when we restrict the sphere of decision-making to the clinician faced with a sick individual, the definition of happiness remains a problem.

Children with acute leukaemia can now survive up to three years or more, but, in the terminal stages the consultant physician may wish to discontinue further treatment. During the patient's frequent admissions a relationship is formed between the staff and the patient's parents, who may often require a good deal of emotional support. It is nearly always the wish of the parents that their child should continue on transfusions and drugs right up to the time of death. We know this is because the parents cannot accept the inevitable, but should we tell them that their reaction is a selfish one, in no way aiding their child's suffering? Or are we wrong to give up hope and 'cease to strive to keep alive'?

In hospital X one of the surgeons carries out an increasing

amount of work of a general nature in major surgery of the head and neck. Patients referred to him suffer from cancer and some are over seventy years of age. The operations invariably include a tracheostomy, are often very disfiguring and result in the patients being unable to speak, eat or drink for the first few days afterwards. Recovery is very prolonged and a great deal of emotional support is required. From time to time members of the nursing staff are very distressed because they feel that it would sometimes be kinder not to operate, but merely to give sedatives. They feel that the older patients would end their days more comfortably in this way, and relatives would not be so upset. Free discussion between the surgeon and the nursing staff on the issue has shown how opinions can vary about what is 'doing the best for the patient'.

These two examples illustrate two well-known, but nonetheless important aspects of clinical practice: the disability of the patient cannot be viewed in isolation from the patient seen as a whole person; and the patient must not be treated in isolation from his relationship to others. The question of 'what is best for the patient' is thus much wider than the question of removing certain disabilities. It involves the assessment of the effect of treatment, or lack of treatment, on the quality of his life and on the lives of those who are closest to him. Of course, there are many situations in which no doubt exists about the best course of action. Doctors do not need to consider the life-situation of a patient in order to decide to alleviate severe pain or to operate on a ruptured appendix or to arrest the course of an infectious illness. In other situations, however, the balancing of one pain against another and the assessment of what will be least distressing to the patient and his relatives are essential components of the decision.

For these reasons medical and nursing staff often find themselves in the situation of trying to define and predict happiness. Does Mill's theory help in the decisions to be taken? It is difficult to see how it does, with the little help it gives in weighing values and obligations. Is there more happiness in dying peacefully than in striving to the end for survival and recovery? Should the effect of a clinical decision on the state of mind of relatives and nursing staff be taken into account at all? Doctors and nurses have to find answers to these questions, and in doing so they are deciding about the potential happiness of others, but it is doubtful whether the concept of quality of happiness will be of much help to them. We simply do not know from Mill's utilitarianism whether 'keeping alive at all costs' is an absolute obligation and whether the happiness of the patient is the only happiness we should consider. We can underline this difficulty by making up an extreme example. Let us suppose that we could keep a patient alive only at a prohibitive cost to his family. Giving the treatment would result in the patient's wife being forced to take employment, leaving younger children at home. One of the older children will have to terminate studies in order to work also. The strain of the situation seems to be adversely affecting the wife's psychological health, yet without the treatment the patient will not survive. Assuming that there is no solution to the problem from outside financial aid, how do we weigh the various amounts of happiness and unhappiness involved? The notion of 'quality of happiness' seems of little or no use in such a situation. What we need to know is where the overriding obligations lie.

We have now seen that, even in the case of the individual clinical decision, the greatest happiness principle does not apply easily because of its vagueness of definition. This is the first major practical difficulty in Mill's philosophy. We shall now look at a second practical problem—that of predicting happiness—but first it must be stressed that we have not yet shown Mill's account to be an incorrect analysis of the meaning of words like 'good' and 'ought'. We have only shown that it does not help in solving specific moral dilemmas. It might still be correct in a formal sense to say that good means 'promoting the greatest happiness', even although the greatest happiness is not easy to define or measure. That is a question to be considered later.

## Predicting Happiness

Even if we suppose that we could solve the difficulty of defining and assessing happiness, a further problem will confront us. How are we to know which courses of action will result in the promotion of the greatest happiness? The following example illustrates how difficult it can be to anticipate the consequences of our decisions:

A doctor volunteered to be a donor for a fellow practitioner who was dying from chronic renal failure. Although he hardly knew the recipient, the doctor felt that he would like to assist a fellow member of his profession, and he did not anticipate any insuperable difficulties resulting from the operation. Unfortunately the recipient died shortly after the operation and the donor's health was affected for some time, resulting in some financial difficulties for his family. The donor felt considerable regret at the decision he had taken, realising that he had not discussed it fully with his wife, who had not really wanted him to undergo the risks. He was also embittered by the discovery that the recipient's widow had remarried and showed no interest in keeping contact with his family.

This kind of unfortunate sequence of consequences is frequently used by opponents of the greatest happiness theory to draw the moral that 'virtue has its own reward', and that it is hopeless to base morality on the improbabilities of happiness. Defenders of the theory, however, are not so easily discouraged. The morality of actions, they argue, must be measured by *intended* consequences, not actual consequences. In the example cited, the donor *intended* to save the life of the recipient without causing undue risk to himself or his family. The facts that the recipient died, his own family suffered and the recipient's wife seemed to lack gratitude, do not take away from the rightness of his intention to promote the general happiness.

There are other cases, however, when the uncertainty of consequences is so great that it is hard to see how we are to make a responsible estimate of probable happiness in order to intend it:

A woman in her early twenties had suffered from a disabling psychotic illness from childhood. Treatment with modern drugs had produced an improvement, relieving her symptoms and allowing her to participate to a greater extent in activities and derive more enjoyment from life. A drug trial was being set up with a recently developed drug and it was decided to include this patient in the experimental group. It was not known whether the drug would effect a further improvement, have no effect or even have an adverse effect, which might not be able to be overcome by reversion to the former drug. Was the risk worth taking? And for what reasons should the risk be taken—because the drug might cause even more improvement in the patient's illness? or because, whatever the effects on this patient, more would be learned about the drug for the benefit of others?

To say that the researchers must intend *both* to give benefit to the patient and to gain fresh knowledge about the effect of the drug sounds a little hollow in a situation in which it is not really known whether both consequences are likely. In terms of happy consequences it will only be known afterwards whether the risk was worth taking. A similar kind of problem in prediction occurs in situations of emergency when decisions have to be taken at high speed, with no time to weigh up imponderables. The technique of resuscitation is a prime example of this kind of need for rapid decision in medical care. The following cases illustrate the difficulties involved:

Mrs A, a thin little woman aged 56 years, was admitted to a surgical ward with the diagnosis of fractured shaft of femur (pathological). Since she had had cancer of the breast some years previously it was assumed that the fracture was due to a secondary deposit in her femur. On examination it was found that she had a tumour, possibly malignant, in her thyroid. Her chances of survival seemed very slender and all that could be anticipated was an increase in pain and disability. She herself seemed quite unaware of the seriousness of her condition, and was always bright and cheerful, her only complaint being a difficulty in swallowing. One afternoon in the week following treatment for the fracture, she suddenly choked when having a drink, her breathing became obstructed and her heart stopped beating. The Senior Registrar who was on the ward at the time, immediately attempted resuscitation by closed methods, and eventually, after carrying out a tracheostomy and opening her chest in order to stimulate the heart manually was successful in bringing her back to life. Many of the staff were critical of this action. Should the patient have been saved, they asked, only to have her agony prolonged? Yet the registrar's prompt intervention meant that Mrs A was able to go home eventually and have a few happy weeks with her husband and daughter. She lived for nine months after her life had been saved by resuscitation.

Mr X was admitted to an accident-emergency department after being pinned underneath a lorry of bricks. He had suffered a fracture dislocation of his cervical vertebrae and was quadriplegic. He was having to use his diaphragm to assist his breathing and his chances of recovery seemed in considerable doubt. Immediate treatment consisted of an intravenous transfusion, a reduction of the fracture dislocation and the application of traction. Early the following morning Mr X's breathing became very laboured and it was decided to perform a tracheostomy, but before this could be carried out he had a cardiac arrest. Without further thought, the

anaesthetist, who was present for the operation, resuscitated
him. The surgeon in charge, who had many years of experience, passed the comment: 'We might live to regret this.'
Mr X never recovered any movement. He failed to accept his
condition and became more morbid as the days went on. He
had to be fed, washed, turned at two-hourly intervals and
was completely unable to do anything for himself. He developed chest and urinary complications; and poor circulation, causing areas of necrosis to form in his tissues, added
to his troubles. The ward staff felt sorry for the relatives in
such a situation, but were quite shocked when they asked the
surgeon to give Mr X 'something to expedite his departure',
because they were all tired out and very inconvenienced with
prolonged visiting. This request was, of course, refused by
the surgeon who pointed out that his work was to save life
not destroy it. Mr X lived in misery for a further six months.
We had done what we thought was right, although it proved
to bring great suffering to the patient and his family. Would
the same thing be done again? Often there isn't time to think,
but I feel fairly sure the answer is 'yes'.

Here we have two examples of the application of an
emergency life-saving measure in situations in which there
was no possibility of calculating consequences. Since any
delay in the institution of resuscitation procedures can
result in brain damage through anoxia, split second decisions have to be taken. In both cases the doctors concerned
acted on the principle that a life had to be saved, without
stopping to estimate whether happy or painful consequences
would follow from their action. Of what possible use can
the Greatest Happiness Principle be in such situations?

Utilitarian philosophers answer this kind of problem
by distinguishing between *primary* and *secondary* principles.
Most of the time, they admit, we do not stop to work out
the consequences of our actions. We rely on a set of
secondary principles concerned with respect for life, keeping
promises, paying debts, acting honestly, etc., which help us
through the day-to-day decisions of life. In an emergency

situation these secondary principles based on the experience of many generations and many different societies, will guide our decision-making. The use of such principles, however, does not disprove the validity of the greatest happiness principle, which (the utilitarians believe) is the *primary* principle of morality upon which the secondary principles have been based. Rules like the one enjoining us to respect life have been formulated because following them is the best way of ensuring that the greatest happiness will result. Therefore it does not matter that a doctor has no time to predict the consequences of resuscitating a patient. By resuscitating he is following the secondary principle of saving human life whenever possible, and following this principle is a way of safeguarding happiness generally.

Yet, as the cases we have used illustrate, following the secondary principle of saving a life if it is within your power to do so does *not* always result in the promotion of the greatest happiness. In the case of Mr X nothing but misery seems to have been created for all concerned, whilst the case of Mrs A is one in which the happiness of the consequences was at least arguable. Despite this, the staff concerned in these incidents felt that, confronted with a similar choice in the future, they would still make every attempt to resuscitate. (As one of the nurses involved in the incident with Mrs A pointed out, they felt unable to stand back and allow her to die when they knew the procedures for restoring life.) Thus it seems to make much more sense to say that resuscitation is carried out because there is a primary moral obligation to save life, not because consequences of one kind or another are expected if the life is saved.

There is a final line of defence available to the utilitarians against this kind of attack. They can adopt a form of the theory known as *rule*-utilitarianism (as distinct from *act*-utilitarianism). The rule-utilitarian concedes that there are some instances of following secondary principles which do not promote the general happiness. (Restoring Mr X to life would be an example of this.) But, although particular acts in accordance with the rules may fail to produce happiness, it is still necessary for the general well-being of a society that there should be such rules and that they should be consistently obeyed. A society whose members only obeyed rules about keeping promises, saving life or respecting property when they were sure it would promote the general happiness to do so, would be a very insecure one. Therefore conformity to rules is necessary for happiness. There is, however, the argument goes on, nothing absolute or unchangeable about the rules which a society adopts. If following a particular rule over a large number of instances seems to cause more pain than happiness, then the rule will be changed for one which is more useful. The only points that have to be safeguarded are that everyone is aware of the alteration in the rule and that the new rule can be seen to be likely to increase the general welfare of the society.

This modified form of utilitarianism seems to harmonise well with the kind of discussion which has developed about the rights and wrongs of resuscitation. Efforts to reach an agreed policy on this in hospitals or treatment units have had to avoid two extremes: on the one hand the view that one must resuscitate under all circumstances, however poor the prognosis of the patient; and on the other, the attempt to categorise whole classes of patient (for example those over a certain age) as 'not to be resuscitated'. The only workable policy seems to be one in which decisions are taken *in advance* about each individual patient on the general principle that it is better to attempt to restore life *unless* the consequences for the patient will be no more than a prolongation of irreversible suffering. The application of the same principle leads to rules about not attempting resuscitation if there has been a time lapse long enough to cause extensive brain damage. This kind of policymaking illustrates the importance of having rules which are weighted toward the preservation of life, but which are flexible enough to ensure that following them will result (for the most part) in relieving suffering also. It is precisely this approach to secondary principles which the rule-utilitarian is advocating.

Thus it seems that, with some theoretical reformulations, utilitarianism is able to withstand the problem of the uncertainty of the consequences of particular actions. This gap is filled by moral rules, or secondary principles, which ultimately depend on the primary principle of the greatest happiness of the greatest number. But in the course of this discussion a more fundamental question has begun to take shape. Is it true to say that all moral rules are ultimately dependent on the greatest happiness principle? Is it because of the effect on general happiness that a doctor has a pressing obligation to restore life in a patient whose heart has stopped, unless there are very good reasons against it? Or are there arguments of a different kind which make this kind of action morally binding, whatever the effect on the general well-being? It seems possible that attempting to base morality on happiness results in a failure to understand the essential character of moral obligation. This possibility will now be explored by examining the relationship between justice and happiness.

## Justice and Happiness

In order to test whether the utilitarian analysis of morality is a correct one we need to discover whether there are cases in which doing what is right is not the same as promoting the general happiness. The concept of 'justice' seems to contain within it an element of overriding obligation which is not explained simply by pointing to the beneficial effects of acting justly. Why, for example, should we respect the rights of individuals in cases where ignoring these rights would seem to be much more advantageous to society as a whole? Good illustrations of the opposition between respect for individuals and general happiness are to be found in the moral issues arising from the use of patients as subjects for clinical research:

The objective of a drug trial is to establish whether one of a number of drugs can control more effectively than others the symptoms which may manifest themselves in a particular illness. Patients are therefore chosen as subjects because of their display of symptoms, and not necessarily because they need a change in treatment. At one psychiatric hospital in which I worked trials were organised using long-term schizophrenic patients. To obtain an objective result several patients, who were established on a maintenance dose of medication. were 'weaned off' and left without support for two weeks. When the trials commenced one group of patients were given a 'placebo' and another put on the drug being tested. In view of the effect on patients of withdrawing drugs which were proving beneficial and the need to deceive some patients with the use of 'placebo', can such experiments be morally right?

The moral ambiguities in research increase when the procedures being tested are not related to the patient's illness.

During my work in paediatric nursing I have been involved in research designed to assess the effect of a certain type of test on children. Administration of the test involved some discomfort for the patients, and the investigation bore no relation to the condition for which the children had been admitted. Moreover, since the research involved X-ray screening, the patients were being exposed to unnecessary radiation.

Recently the medical profession has discussed very fully moral problems in the use of patients for research projects, and in 1964 the World Medical Association adopted the *Declaration of Helsinki* (see Appendix), which laid down principles upon which experimentation should be conducted. This code drew a fundamental distinction between research which was potentially of value to the patients involved (therapeutic research) and research which was of no therapeutic value to the patients involved (non-therapeutic research). In both cases the Declaration stresses the importance of giving the patient a full explanation and of obtaining his free consent. The necessity for consent is particularly stressed in cases of non-therapeutic research; in such cases the Declaration states: 'The investigator must respect the right of each individual to safeguard his personal integrity, especially if the subject is in a dependent relationship to him'. (For a fuller discussion of this issue *see* Chapter Six.)

Why—we must ask the utilitarian—do we put such a stress on the integrity of the individual in the clinical research situation? After all, research in medicine is aimed at benefiting mankind as a whole; surely then general happiness would be better served by being less scrupulous about the rights of individuals, when insisting on full consent is going to limit the scope of research which can be carried out. It seems that the only reason that we do maintain the importance of the individual is that we feel we have an absolute duty to do so, even in the face of failing to promote the good of the majority.

John Stuart Mill was well aware that this kind of obligation posed a serious problem for his theory (although he was not, of course, familiar with the kind of clinical problems which we have used as examples). In his essay, *Utilitarianism*, he discussed the difficulty under the heading, 'On the Connexion between Justice and Utility'. Why is it, he asked, that we put so much stress on matters like the rights of individuals and the necessity for equality of treatment? His answer was that these moral requirements are more socially useful than any others and that therefore they have a stronger feeling of obligation attached to them. The feeling of obligation he also attempts to explain psychologically by saying that it is the natural feeling of resentment which we would feel if *our* rights were infringed extended to cover *everyone*'s rights by a feeling of sympathy for all men.

This argument of Mill's simply will not hold water, since it fails to explain why an equitable treatment of every individual should be more socially useful than a policy which disregards the rights of some individuals in order greatly to increase the welfare of the majority in the society. Experiments conducted on the mentally subnormal and the inmates of concentration camps in Nazi Germany were, it was claimed by the doctors involved, aimed at the benefit of the rest of humanity. Mill's psychological argument about universalised resentment against infringement of rights is no defence at all against this kind of attitude. Such feelings, the Nazi experimenter would say, must be brushed aside. Why should a few Jews or a few imbeciles be of any consequence?

Of course Mill and his fellow utilitarians would be horrified by this use of their theory. All their energies were devoted toward eradicating social injustice and extending the rights of the individual. But they seem to have been assuming certain moral values to be essential which could never be justified by happiness alone. Even the more subtle argument about the need for consistent rules in order to have a secure society (to which we referred in the previous section) will not prove that the rules have to be perfectly fair in order to be socially useful. If the greatest number of people in a society are of normal intelligence, there would be no reason for them to feel insecure in a society which ignored the rights of the mentally subnormal, since this kind of discrimination will not affect them in any way. Similarly a society whose members were nearly all of one skin colour could feel quite secure with laws which restricted the rights of people of a different skin colour, since there would be no possibility of these laws ever affecting the majority's well-being. Equality of treatment is only important for general happiness in areas of justice in which anyone might at one time or another be the one suffering the injustice.

The flaw in the utilitarian argument about justice lies in a confusion between what is useful or advantageous to the majority and what we feel all men ought to value. Mill is clearly of the opinion that all men ought to value freedom and equality, even if it is a little to the disadvantage of the majority to treat everyone with perfect justice. It is only clouding the issue to keep asserting that justice and social utility are the same. This is really making a contradictory statement: that it is advantageous to the majority to support that which may be disadvantageous to them. Logic is better served by saying that, although treating every individual justly usually does benefit the society as a whole, even in cases in which there is no social benefit justice must still be done. To put it in these terms is to say that respect for the rights of the individual is a more fundamental moral value than the happiness of the majority, and therefore to reject Greatest Happiness Theory.

We have now questioned the adequacy of the concept of happiness to serve as the central point of moral decision, both on practical and theoretical grounds. However, the importance of utilitarianism can be seen from the amount of discussion which has been required in order to reach these conclusions. In a great many of the dilemmas of personal and social morality the criterion of general happiness is a good corrective to personal bias and idealistic mouthing of principles. Medical care, in particular, rests very heavily on the sustained and dedicated opposition to pain and on the determination to attack those barriers to happiness in our societies which will yield to the application of scientific research and therapeutic skill. The Greatest Happiness of the Greatest Number is a valuable description of part of the aim of moral action, but there are occasions when it is not precise enough in its definition of moral value to provide a satisfactory analysis of the dilemmas men face.

## REFERENCES

Eckstein, H. (1964). *The English Health Service.* Cambridge: Harvard U.P.

Flinn, M. W. (1968). *Public Health Reform in Britain.* London: Macmillan.

Longmate, N. (1966). *King Cholera.* London: Hamish Hamilton.

Medical Services Review Committee (1958). *A Review of Medical Services in Great Britain.*

Mill, J. S. (1859). *On Liberty.* (Rationalist Press Reprint, 1903.) London: Watts.

Mill, J. S. (1867). *Utilitarianism,* 3rd ed. London: Longmans.

Ross, J. S. (1952). *The National Health Service in Great Britain.* Oxford University Press.

Thomson, D. (1950). *England in the Nineteenth Century.* London: Penguin.

Willcocks, A. J. (1967). *The Creation of the National Health Service.* London: Routledge and Kegan Paul.

# CHAPTER FOUR

# Rules and Situations

If we abandon the appeal to the benefit of the majority as a way of settling disputes in morality, we are brought rapidly to the point of searching for some set of absolute or fundamental values, which will clearly and unambiguously inform our choices and decisions in any given situation. Such a quest for absolutes is based on the conviction that morality has a universal aspect to it which is not subject to the vagaries of individual inclination or social necessity. The absolutist point of view in ethical theory is well represented by the following quotation from a textbook of nursing ethics:

'Morality is not a matter of current opinions or actions of the majority; it is not a matter of what is useful at the moment, of a spirit of altruism, of expediency, of feeling. It is not a matter of social usefulness; ...
  'Morality is intrinsic, objective and unchanging.'
(Hayes et al., 1964, p. 11.)

Ethical theories of this type can take several forms. In this chapter we shall be concerned with that form which gives a central place to the concept of *moral law*. In the chapter which follows we shall examine theories based on the ideal of *respect for persons*.


## Law and Human Nature

The experience of acting according to a set of laws, rules

or principles is such a familiar one that most of the time it goes unnoticed by us. Rule following, much of it habitual and unquestioned, characterises a high proportion of our daily activity. Our behaviour is confined within the limits of the socially acceptable, the legally sanctioned and the routines of personal preference and conviction. Thus most of our actions are quite predictable to anyone who knows our character and our social background. Sometimes, of course, we do deviate from the rules, but such deviance merely serves to underline the predictability of most of our actions most of the time. But the interest of the ethical theorist is aroused when the question is asked whether there are circumstances in which the rules which define our habitual ways of acting *ought* to be broken. Little difficulty arises in the case of social conventions. It is easy to imagine situations in which they must be disregarded in order to act effectively and honestly. Often the unconventional person is struggling to reach personal and interpersonal realities beneath the veneer of politeness which characterizes so much social interaction. With less certainty we can identify limitations to legal prohibitions. In many historical instances laws have been enacted by particular states, which individuals have felt compelled to disobey on grounds of conscience. (For example, segregationist laws, or laws forbidding political demonstrations.) But the debate begins in earnest when we come to principles of morality. Do they have a binding character which permits of no exceptions, or are there occasions when they too *ought* to be disregarded?

The following description of an elaborate and deliberate act of deception illustrates the point at issue:

The mother of a subnormal child was forbidden by her husband to see her baby after he had been admitted to hospital for long-term care. She kept up a lively and optimistic correspondence with the staff about him, writing of her hopes of his attending school. She was clearly unaware of the fact that the boy had deteriorated considerably since admission and was bedfast. After a number of years it transpired that the mother was dying of disseminated sclerosis, and she asked to be allowed to see her son. The husband came to discuss the matter with me and convinced me that it would greatly upset his wife to see the boy as he really was, because he had given her a completely false picture of how he was getting on. Knowing that the woman was dying, I decided to select a patient of the same age and colouring and allow him to the visit as her son. Two days after the visit the mother died. I feel that what I did was an act of benevolence, and although it was deception I don't think it was wrong. I was told that the mother was made very happy by the visit. The husband, I feel, was doing what he could in the situation he had created. The substitute 'son' was himself of subnormal intelligence and obviously enjoyed the ride and all the attention he received. The real son was deprived of nothing, since he was incapable of recognising his parents in any case.

In this example we have the case of an individual, who would normally regard deception as morally wrong, considering that the situation in which he found himself obliged him to break the rule that one should not deceive others. Many moralists would argue that his reasoning in this situation was quite misguided. Deception, they would assert, should never be knowingly practised, with whatever good intentions, since the principle forbidding deception can only retain its force by being applied to *all* cases. If an exception is allowed in one case, it may equally be argued for in countless others, until morality becomes merely a matter of personal opinion and is drained of all objectivity. It is the theories upon which such an absolutist view of moral principles is based that we now wish to examine.

The assigning of an objective character to moral principles has found its fullest elaboration in the doctrine of *natural law*, which has roots as far back as the Greek school of philosophy known as Stoicism. The Stoics maintained that there was a Divine Law dwelling in the universe, which could be discerned by any human being through the exercise of reason. The commands of such a law ensured that each individual would live in disciplined conformity to the rational, disregarding any considerations of emotion or desire. The Stoic philosophy had a profound effect on Roman civilisation at the beginning of the Imperial period. Thus in the writings of the Roman philosopher and jurist, Cicero, we find a full description of the doctrine of natural law:

True law is right reason in agreement with Nature; it is of universal application, unchanging and everlasting; it summons to duty by its commands, and averts wrong-doing by its prohibitions ... It is a sin to try to alter this law, nor is it allowable to attempt to repeal any part of it, and it is impossible to try to abolish it entirely ... And there will not be different laws at Rome and at Athens, or different laws now and in the future, but one eternal, and unchangeable law will be valid for all nations and for all times and there will be one master and one ruler, that is, God, over us all, for He is the author of this law, its promulgator, and its enforcing judge.

(*De Republica*, III, xxii, 33.)

This concept of a universal immanent law of nature was finally deeply imprinted upon all Western theological, philosophical and legal theory by the mediaeval theologian Thomas Aquinas, whose *Summa Theologica* laid out a totally comprehensive system of relationships between the natural and the supernatural. The Thomist system of thought defined the terms of intellectual debate at least until the time of the Renaissance, and it remains to the present day the base-line for all expositions of Roman Catholic moral theology. Two features of the natural law approach to ethics merit special attention: its use of the term 'natural'; and its grounding of morality in statements of religious faith.

## Natural and Unnatural

Fundamental to the concept of natural law is the distinction between natural and unnatural, which in turn depends on the view that all things serve a certain end or purpose. Natural law is regarded as that which delineates the true, or divinely intended end of man. It sets the pattern of the authentically human, which may differ considerably from the way in which most human beings behave (Vann, 1965, p. 75).

What characterises the 'authentically human'? Aquinas' exposition of this is expressed by the first principle of the natural law: 'good is to be done and promoted, and evil is to be avoided'. This principle sounds rather like a statement of the obvious, a mere repetition of part of the meaning of the terms 'good' and 'evil', but its association with the term 'natural' is important. For this approach to ethics, morality *fulfills human beings' potentialities*. Man becomes fully man through moral action: he destroys himself through pursuing evil. Such a view has been supported by many modern writers, whose approach is far removed from that of Thomist moral theology (e.g. Waddington, 1942; Rogers, 1961).

Things begin to get more difficult, however, when we look beyond the broad statement that morality is that which helps man to be more truly himself, to specific statements about which acts are good or natural and which acts are evil or unnatural. Are suicide, birth control, and sexual intercourse outside marriage unnatural in this sense? Roman Catholic moral theologians argue that they are, seeing them as violations of the natural law, whose cardinal principles are self-preservation, procreation and intellectual and moral development (Welty, 1960, p. 232). Yet, for the Stoics of ancient Rome suicide could be the final act of rationality, an authentically human gesture; some modern Catholic writers have argued that birth control could be a more responsibly human act than the refusal to plan parenthood (e.g. St. John-Stevas, 1971); and in some recent statements by Protestant writers extramarital sexual relationships have not been seen to be in all circumstances morally wrong (Heron, 1963; British Council of Churches Working Party, 1966).

We are not concerned at this stage to argue the question of whether suicide, contraception and sexual intercourse outside marriage are, or are not, morally wrong, but merely to demonstrate that this question cannot be settled by a simple appeal to the concept of 'natural'. Despite the fact that some writers seem to think that the principles of the natural law are as self-evident as the axioms of mathematics (Marshall, 1960, p. 4), any specific formulations of it which are put forward by one moral theorist are likely to be questioned by many other moral theorists, who show every sign of possessing normal reasoning powers.

There is a straightforward logical reason for this lack of agreement about the reference of the term 'natural': it is that the term is being used *evaluatively,* not merely *descriptively.* Since it is saying what man ought to be, not merely what man is, its reference is not open to simple testing by observations of the way people actually behave. Rather its application depends on the convictions of the user about the true nature and destiny of man. These convictions may or may not be shared by other rational beings. Thus we are quickly brought to the other feature of natural law theory: its grounding in religious belief.

## Faith and Rationality

In the Thomist exposition of natural law revelation and reason are regarded as complementary. God, the ultimate source of all law, has implanted in man the light of reason and by this means all men, whether believers or unbelievers, are able to know the difference between good and evil. In addition, God has revealed his will to men through the divine law of the Old and New Testaments, which harmonises perfectly with the natural law. God has entrusted to the Church the absolute authority to make known and to interpret the natural law with infallible certainty (Welty, 1960, p. 244), and to demonstrate its harmony with revealed law.

Such an account of natural law appears to see faith and rationality as two independent streams flowing from the same source, but without contamination, as it were, of the one by the other. This point of view can be maintained only by arguing that all those rational individuals who disagree with the Roman Catholic Church's interpretations of the natural law do so because their reasoning is confused—the complexity of the situations they are in, or their personal prejudices, having clouded their judgment. Such a point of view cannot be refuted, since all evidence brought forward to show divergences from the Catholic interpretations of the moral law by reasoning individuals are automatically refuted by the basic conviction that the Church cannot err in its teaching. The Roman Catholic position is perfectly consistent, provided one accepts the first premise: that through the church the will of God is infallibly known.

Another interpretation of the situation, however, is one which sees faith and reason as inextricably bound together in any attempt to formulate moral absolutes. In this view rationality is regarded as an intellectual tool which functions to test the validity of arguments, once certain assumptions are granted. These assumptions are not themselves open to demonstration by reasoned argument, but are the starting points from which reasoning begins. At the basis of moral reasoning, then, is a set of faith statements rather than a set of fact statements. These faith statements vary from individual to individual and from culture to culture and are intimately connected to the fabric of religious belief interwoven between individuals and groups at different times and places. Such a view (as the Roman Catholic moral theologian would be quick to point out) introduces an element of relativity to moral principles. It does not necessarily mean, however, that all moral assertions are reduced to matters of personal opinion. To point to the non-rational character of basic moral assertions is not the same as saying that it is of no importance what moral opinions an individual has. It is merely questioning the notion that fundamental moral values can be expressed in the form of self-evident rational principles. Whether they can be expressed in any other way which transcends mere personal preference is a question to be explored in the next chapter. For the present the purely negative point has been argued, that an appeal to the 'purely rational' does not solve disagreements in matters of morality. This negative point may be illustrated by the following clinical examples:

A woman was admitted to a maternity ward in the early stages of labour. Prenatal examination had indicated that she was expecting twins. Since she had a very pale appearance a blood count was taken and the haemoglobin level was esti-

mated at only 25 per cent. In view of the likelihood of haemorrhage after delivery the doctor instructed the midwife in
charge to make five pints of blood available. But when the
nurse started to put up the first pint of blood the patient immediately objected, explaining that she was a Jehovah's
Witness, and that her religion forbade her to have a blood
transfusion. The staff tried to argue with her, explaining the
dangers to her babies as well as to herself, if blood were with-
held. Since she remained adamant, her husband was sent for
and the matter discussed with him in the hope that he would
persuade his wife to change her mind. However, he agreed
with her decision, declaring that: 'If God wishes her to die,
she will die, but she will not have another person's blood,
because the law of God forbids it.' In the event the hospital
staff disregarded the patient's wishes at a late stage in delivery,
after she had lost consciousness, and succeeded in delivering
both babies alive, although they were clearly suffering the
effects of placental insufficiency. Despite continued use of
transfusions and attempts at resuscitation the mother died
six hours later.

Anyone not sharing the religious beliefs of the Jehovah's
Witnesses is likely to find the moral convictions of the
parents in this example hard to comprehend. Yet there
was simply no way for the staff to reason with them, since
in their estimation the accepting of a blood transfusion
was an evil greater than that of risking the lives of their
unborn children. These lives, they believed, and the life of
the mother, must be left in the hands of God. The second
case illustrates the logical outcome of a different set of
religious convictions. In this instance a Catholic patient
based her decision on her belief in the priority of the life
of a fetus over her own life.

A Roman Catholic patient in her early forties was admitted
to a gynaecological ward in the third month of her pregnancy. She already had a large family and had in recent years
been suffering from chronic heart disease. The consultant in
charge of the ward was very concerned about the potential

effect of a continuation of the pregnancy on her health, even with in-patient care up to the time of delivery. He considered it most likely that her life would be jeopardised by the strains of childbirth, or that her health would be so badly affected that she would be unable to care for the other children. On these grounds he tried to persuade the patient to have an abortion and so did several of the nursing staff. The patient, however, refused to consider it, feeling that she would rather risk her own life than live with the death of an innocent child on her conscience. A few weeks later she miscarried and the dilemma was thus avoided.

As with the first case, there was no likelihood of arguing the patient out of her decision without making her abandon her religious faith. To the staff not sharing her convictions her responsibilities as a mother seemed to carry a greater weight than the continued existence of an unborn fetus. But to the patient that fetus had an immortal soul, a destiny in the eyes of God, which she dared not interfere with. Both cases illustrate the rationality of moral principles, *given* a set of beliefs about the nature and destiny of human life. The rationality provides some common ground for discussion: but on matters of belief individuals notoriously differ.

We have argued that, in view of its interdependence with religious belief, the concept of natural law does not provide an adequate foundation for a universally acknowledged set of moral rules. Yet we have not yet shown that any analysis of morality in terms of law is bound to be unsatisfactory. What will happen if we abandon the evaluative term 'natural' and look simply at the formal notion of law? Within such a notion there may be contained the definitive character of morality, even if the filling in of the abstract form is fraught with uncertainty and ambiguity. We can explore this possibility by looking at the philosophy of **Immanuel Kant** (1724–1804), who attempted to argue toward an account of moral law through an analysis of the everyday notion of doing one's duty.

## Duty and the Moral Law

One could summarise Kant's approach (in terms of which he himself would hardly approve!) by saying that he believed that the guts of morality were to be found in the experience of doing one's duty for duty's sake and for no other reason. Often, Kant conceded, one's duty might coincide with that which brings pleasure or with that which one feels inclined to do in any case, but the test cases arise when we find duty to be in conflict with our desires or to threaten unhappy consequences for ourselves or others. In such cases we realise that what is required of us is to persevere in duty, irrespective of our desires or of the foreseeable consequences.

Having dispensed with the quest for happiness or satisfaction as a criterion of the morally right, Kant goes on to subject the notion of duty to further scrutiny. He observes that the obligation which duty conveys can be seen to be cast in the form of a command or of a prohibition ('Do X' or 'Shun Y'). Thus underlying the notion of duty is the concept of 'imperatives' or 'practical principles', which prescribe and proscribe actions. Two types of imperative can be identified: (1) *Hypothetical imperatives*, which prescribe the type of action required to attain a certain end. (For example: 'If you want to maintain your health, then you must take regular exercise'.); and (2) *Categorical imperatives* which state unconditionally which actions must be done or not done. (Kant gives as an example of this the command: 'Do not make deceitful promises'.) It is the second type of imperative—the categorical—that underlies the notion of duty and, therefore, is at the foundation of morality.

The final stage of Kant's analysis is an explanation of what it is about categorical imperatives that gives them their unconditional character. He offers a set of inter-related answers to this question, each to be regarded as an alternative formulation of *the* categorical imperative (or *the* moral law). Firstly, he argues that the inescapable character of moral rules is based on their capacity to apply with equal force to any being (be he man or angel) who possesses rationality. This he conveys in the formula: 'So act that the maxim of your action can become a universal law for all rational beings'. Secondly, he argues that moral rules derive their obligation from their capacity to function as laws of nature, that is to say, to fit into a system of rational laws describing the nature of things. ('Act as if the maxim of your action were to become by your will a universal law of nature.') Thirdly, he argues that the obligation derives from the capacity of moral values to create a community of moral agents. ('So act as to treat humanity, whether in your own person or in that of any other, in every case as an end, never as a mere means.')

Kant's analysis is couched in such abstract terms that it is difficult to keep clearly in view what he has in fact asserted. Putting all the elements together, we seem to arrive at the general statement that the obligatory nature of morality derives from the capacity of moral rules to function as the freely chosen principles of a harmoniously self-governing group of rational beings who are themselves a part of a rational universe. The boundaries of such a group must be able to be extended to include all rational beings, otherwise the rules adopted will not retain their binding character. Thus if any particular maxim is proposed, it can only be accepted as a genuinely moral rule if it fulfills all the conditions laid down—universally applicable, coherent with a rational system of nature, capable of being freely adopted by a community of rational beings.

Now let us try to see how Kant's theory deals with specific situations, using first one of his own examples and then an example from modern medicine.

Kant takes the prohibition of suicide as an example of a maxim which commands categorically and is therefore part of the moral law:

'A man reduced to despair by a series of misfortunes feels wearied of life, but is still so far in possession of his reason that he can ask himself whether it would not be contrary to his duty to himself to take his own life. Now he inquires whether the maxim of his action could become a universal law of nature. His maxim is: From self-love I adopt as a principle to shorten my life when its longer duration is likely to bring more evil than satisfaction. It is asked then simply whether this principle founded on self-love can become a universal law of nature. Now we see at once that a system of nature of which it should be a law to destroy life by means of the very feeling whose special nature it is to impel to the improvement of life would contradict itself and therefore could not exist as a system of nature; hence that maxim cannot possibly exist as a universal law of nature, and consequently would be wholly inconsistent with the supreme principle of all duty.' (*Fundamental Principles of the Metaphysic of Morals*, p. 39.)

We see in this quotation Kant's use of the logical principle of non-contradiction (you cannot use the urge to *improve* life to *destroy* life) as a test of whether the maxim conforms to universal law. We shall examine this kind of test in more detail shortly, but first we should notice that exactly the same form of argument which Kant uses against suicide would apply to support the medical decisions taken in the following case, which appeared in the

*British Medical Journal* under the title, 'Not Allowed to Die':

A doctor aged sixty-eight was admitted to an overseas hospital after a barium meal had shown a large carcinoma of the stomach. He had retired from practice five years earlier, after severe myocardial infarction had left his exercise tolerance considerably reduced. The early symptoms of the carcinoma were mistakenly thought to be due to myocardial ischaemia. By the time the possibility of carcinoma was first considered the disease was already far advanced; laparotomy showed extensive metastatic involvement of the abdominal lymph nodes and liver. Palliative gastrectomy was performed with the object of preventing perforation of the primary tumour into the peritoneal cavity, which appeared to the surgeon to be imminent. Histological examination showed the growth to be an anaplastic primary adeno-carcinoma. There was clinical and radiological evidence of secondary deposits in the low thoracic and lumbar vertebrae.

The patient was told of the findings and fully understood their import. In spite of increasingly large doses of pethidine, and of morphine at night, he suffered constantly with severe abdominal pain and pain resulting from compression of spinal nerves by tumour deposits.

On the tenth day after the gastrectomy the patient collapsed with classic manifestations of massive pulmonary embolism. Pulmonary embolectomy was successfully performed in the ward by a registrar. When the patient had recovered sufficiently he expressed his appreciation of the good intention and skill of his young colleague. At the same time he asked that if he had a further cardiovascular collapse no steps should be taken to prolong his life, for the pain of his cancer was now more than he could needlessly continue to endure. He himself wrote a note to this effect in his case records, and the staff of the hospital knew his feelings.

His wish notwithstanding, when the patient collapsed again, two weeks after the embolectomy—this time with acute myocardial infarction and cardiac arrest—he was revived by the hospital's emergency resuscitation team. His heart stopped on four further occasions during that night and each time was restarted artificially. The body then recovered sufficiently to linger for three more weeks but in a decrebrate state, punctuated by episodes of projectile vomiting accompanied by generalised convulsions. Intravenous nourishment was carefully combined with blood transfusion and measures necessary to maintain electrolyte and fluid balance. In addition, antibacterial and antifungal antibiotics were given as prophylaxis against infection particularly pneumonia complicating the tracheotomy that had been performed to ensure a clear airway. On the last day of his illness, preparations were being made for the work of the failing respiratory centre to be given over to an artificial respirator, but the heart finally stopped before this endeavour could be realised.

This case report is submitted for publication without commentary or conclusions, which are left for those who may read it to provide for themselves. (Symmers, 1968, quoted in Smith, H. L., *Ethics and the New Medicine*, p. 133.)

There are of course important differences between this case and Kant's example of the person who contemplates taking his own life, but the *principle* is the same. The patient in the clinical case was, on Kant's analysis, using the urge to improve life (self love) as a basis for asking the medical staff not to preserve it. It would appear that for Kant duty would require perseverance to the bitter end at whatever cost in pain, discomfort and indignity. For this reason alone the Kantian analysis would totally oppose the advocates of voluntary euthanasia, that is those who propose granting to the patient the right to request that his life be ended (*see* Chapter Six).

How useful is Kant's analysis of the fundamental principles of morality? Has its concept of universal law any relevance to the specific dilemmas which confront doctors and nurses? Moral philosophers dislike questions of usefulness or relevance being raised concerning their theories, arguing that their task is merely one of conceptual clarification. In the case of Kant's theory, Duncan (1957) has argued strongly that it is a purely formal analysis of the character or moral obligation and is not intended to provide a way of settling particular moral problems. On this analysis, the categorical imperative in its several formulations defines the conditions necessary for viewing a maxim as morally binding, but does not itself provide the content of a code of morality.

If Duncan's interpretation is correct then we can apply only a negative test on the basis of Kant's theory—one which will clear our actions of personal bias or special pleading insisting that they must be universalisable in order to be morally obligatory—but one which will not be sufficient to delineate the character of the good life to which we should aspire. We can find a use of Kantian philosophy as this kind of negative criterion in M. H. Pappworth's study of clinical research entitled *Human Guinea Pigs*, in which the 'principle of equality' is suggested as a way of testing the morality of any research project. By this principle Pappworth urges the researcher to suppose that he or some person close to him, such as a wife, or son, were the subject on whom the research was to be carried out. If under these circumstances the researcher could genuinely want the research to proceed, then his assertion that no harm will come to the patient is presumably an honest one. Clearly such a test alone is not sufficient to establish whether a given research project ought to be carried out. (Pappworth lists several other criteria which would also have to be satisfied.) Thus as a purely negative criterion—defining the necessary but not sufficient conditions for knowing what our duty is— Kant's analysis is strictly limited in its usefulness. Indeed some critics have argued that it has a potentially harmful effect on the understanding of one's duty by focusing on its purely formal aspect to the detriment of sensitivity to the personal and emotional aspects of moral obligation.

Yet Kant himself appeared to believe that his theory provided far more than negative safeguards (although Duncan may well be right in saying that at this point Kant was guilty of confused thinking). As the quotation from Kant's own writing on the subject of suicide demonstrates, he tried to use the principal of universalisability as a way of establishing the nature of duties towards oneself and others. Moreover, even if this is an aberration from the purity of the Kantian approach perpetrated by its founder, it is an approach which has been shared by moral law theories. It has been typical of such theories, particularly those in the 'natural law' tradition, to develop a complex system of deductive reasoning which allows the application of universal rules of morality to particular situations. We shall, therefore, turn our attention to some of the methods of reasoning, by which such deductions have been carried out in order to determine how far the moral law approach to morality will take us in the definition of specific duties.

## Applying Rules to Cases

The method of reasoning which attempts to apply moral rules to particular cases is correctly described by the term 'casuistry'. This term has fallen into disrepute in modern times, now being used to describe a line of reasoning which is fallacious or in some way suspect. The question of whether casuistic arguments are valid or invalid will be explored in this section through the examination of some of the more commonly used deductive methods. We shall consider first Kant's use of the principle of non-contradiction and then go on to discuss various uses of the distinction between means and ends.

## NON-CONTRADICTION

The logical law of non-contradiction states that proposition cannot be both true and false at the same time. The law can be stated formally as follows: 'If A is true, then not-A is false'. We have just seen that this law is used by Kant to argue that the principle of enhancing life cannot be used as the basis of an argument for destroying it. The difficulty with laws of logic, however, is that they work properly only when one is asserting tautologies (that is, statements which say the same thing twice). Thus, in the case of Kant's example, we can readily agree that it is nonsense to state that the principle of not-destroying life justifies destroying it. However, such a straightforward contradiction is not in fact being asserted by those patients who, in view of their medical condition, rationally contemplate suicide or who wish no further effort to be made to prolong their life. The principle upon which they are basing their decision is that the cessation of life is preferable to its continuation in a form which is destructive of its true character. There is nothing logically contradictory in such an argument, which is stating that one form of not-life (death) is preferable to another form of not-life (a continued biological survival de-humanised by pain or by loss of function). These alternatives have been conveyed in strongly worded phrases by the theologian Joseph Fletcher in an article discussing the morality of euthanasia:

'The classical deathbed scene, with its loving partings and solemn words, is practically a thing of the past. In its stead is a sedated, comatose, betubed object, manipulated and subconscious, if not subhuman.' (Fletcher, 1967, p. 147.)

Fletcher's protest against indignity in death serves to illustrate how ambiguously words like life and death are used when applications of the principle of the sanctity of human life to particular situations are made. In order to make the principle of non-contradiction work in such situations it becomes necessary to assert an identity in the meanings of terms, whose meanings are in fact discrete. (This is known as the fallacy of equivocacy.) Another example of this type of argument is the assertion that all forms of direct abortion are wrong because they entail the murder of an innocent life (see Marshall, 1960; Flood, 1969). This argument depends on equivocacy in the use of the terms 'murder' and 'life'. Murder is the taking of the life of another human being 'with malice aforethought': abortion (as practised under the present law in Great Britain) is the destruction of a fetus in order to save life or prevent suffering. It *may* well be the case that destruction of a fetus is an unjustified form of destruction of a potential person, but the point cannot be proved by supposing that abortion and murder are logically equivalent. The statement that abortion is wrong follows from the statement that murder is wrong *only* if other assumptions are added, such as the belief that the fetus is a full person in the eyes of God and the conviction that the surgeon's intent is malicious. (It should be noted, however, that the common law usage of the term 'malice' means little more than 'deliberate intent'.)

On the basis of these examples, at least, it seems unlikely that the principle of non-contradiction is going to be equal to the task of working out the applications of moral rules to the more complex dilemmas of medical care. It may be a useful principle for preventing individuals from defending their actions by faulty reasoning from premise to conclusion. (The man who argued that stealing was wrong, but there was nothing wrong in riding on a train without paying for a ticket, might well benefit from its application.) It is not so helpful when the applicability of the principle to situations is itself in doubt, or when two or more principles appear to be in contradiction. In matters of life and death the problem is so often one of the uncertainties of definition, or of the necessity to choose the lesser of two evils. When the assigning of moral qualities to actions is rendered ambiguous in this way, an appeal to non-contradiction is of no help.

## MEANS AND ENDS

A second way of relating general moral principles to particular situations is to draw a distinction between the ends to which actions are directed and the means employed to obtain these ends. Three applications of these categories merit attention within the context of medical ethics : (1) Kant's argument that persons must be regarded as *ends in themselves*; (2) the discrimination between types of medical intervention in terms of *ordinary and extraordinary means*; and (3) the method of determining which means are permissible in order to obtain a desired end, known as the *principle of two-fold effect*.

### Ends in Themselves

We owe to Kant a careful analysis of the relationship between moral agents and the means which they employ to achieve their objectives. We have seen that Kant regarded rational beings as possessing a unique capacity to choose for themselves rules for behaviour and to act consistently out of respect for this self-imposed moral law. Kant summarised this description in the phrase 'autonomous' or 'self-legislating' being. In view of this uniqueness, he went on to argue, it can never be morally permissible for one moral agent to use another as a mere means, that is in a way that deprives him or his capacity to choose. Human beings have to use one another in order to achieve objectives, but such a use is only justified when the person used freely chooses to act in this way. He must always remain an 'end in himself'.

One can see applications of this Kantian principle more easily than was possible in the case of the law of non-contradiction. For example, it enables us to lay down clear guide-lines for the relationship between patients and staff in hospitals. Doctor-patient and nurse-patient relationships break through the bounds of morality when one or other party is robbed of his autonomy. Doctors and nurses are used as a means toward recovery by patients, but this can never mean that the patient can demand anything he chooses of the staff. The patient can only expect the fulfilment of those ends to which those who attend him are also committed. (The 'conscience clause' in the Abortion Act of 1967 demonstrates this principle. Should voluntary euthanasia ever be legalised, similar safeguards would be essential. No doctor could be required to assume the function of executioner.) The same principle applies to treatment of patients by staff. Except in certain certifiable conditions, participation in treatment by patients depends wholly on their consent. (For this reason, consent is crucial in situations in which the treatment 'contract' no longer applies, e.g. the use of patients for clinical demonstrations or in research projects of no direct benefit to them.)

Thus the principle of treating persons as ends in themselves does seem to find direct application to clinical situations. Its use as a fundamental principle of morality will be explored further in the next chapter under the heading of 'respect for persons'.

## Ordinary and Extra-ordinary Means

The application of the doctrine of natural law to clinical medical practice has involved the drawing of a distinction between ordinary and extra-ordinary means. As we observed earlier in the chapter, the preservation of life has been regarded as a fundamental principle of the natural law and thus suicide and deliberately causing the death of another are seen to be violations of these principles. Does it then follow that a patient is under an obligation to take all means available for the preservation of his life, in order to avoid committing suicide?; and is a doctor under an obligation to employ all such means if they are at his disposal, in order to avoid committing murder? The concept of 'extra-ordinary means' relieves doctors and patients of such obligations, arising from the principle of the sanctity of life, by arguing that there is no absolute obligation to employ any means which will cause an intolerable burden to the patient or his relatives (see Pius XII, 1957). What constitutes an 'intolerable burden' depends on the circumstances of the patient, the degree of development of the particular medication or surgical procedure and the cost and availability of the treatment proposed. Thus penicillin might have been regarded as an extra-ordinary means at one time because of cost and uncertainty of its effect, but now it is clearly an ordinary means of combating infection. Haemodialysis and organ transplantation appear to fall into the extra-ordinary category at present because of the high cost of the former and the uncertain success rate of the latter, but in the future they may become routine and relatively inexpensive procedures.

It will be observed that this principle provides only a rough and ready guide for the application of the obligation to preserve life. What constitutes an intolerable burden to patient or relatives is a matter of the opinion of the individual clinician, as the following case illustrates:

A baby was born with such severe congenital abnormalities that the surgeon called in to attend to the case decided that it was simply inoperable. He let it be known to the staff involved that his attitude was: 'Thou shalt not kill, but needst not strive officiously to keep alive.' The nursing staff endeavoured to make the baby as comfortable as possible, but were uncertain what to do when the baby's colour became poor. Should they administer oxygen? Should they call the surgeon in charge, knowing that his attitude was one of not making an effort to save the child's life? What would the attitude of the medical and nursing staff have been had the child's parents been present when its condition worsened? Would they have felt an obligation to take more definite action in order to make the parents feel that something was being done?

In terms of cost and availability, the administration of oxygen is certainly to be regarded as an ordinary means, whilst the decision not to operate might be regarded as a decision not to impose a useless and unnecessary burden on patient and relatives. Yet not allowing so damaged a baby to die by giving oxygen might equally be regarded as an intolerable burden to impose on baby and parents. It was not a difference in the quality of the means to be employed that doctor and nurse had to make up their minds about, but rather the character of the *end* they were achieving either by keeping the baby alive or by allowing it to die. The distinction between ordinary and extra-ordinary means ceases to be helpful when really difficult decisions about the quality of life have to be taken. In such situations—as we shall be arguing in more detail in the next section—it is the end sought which determines the character of the treatment employed.

## Two-fold Effect

The final elaboration of the means-ends distinction is one which is designed to cope with situations in which the attempt to achieve one desirable end seems inevitably to involve failing to achieve another. A doctor wishing to alleviate pain in a terminally ill patient uses opiates to which he will become addicted and which will eventually shorten his life. A critically ill patient whose continued survival depends on his hope of recovery is lied to by those around him when he asks about his illness. A leucotomy is performed on a psychiatric patient which diminishes his distressing symptoms but at the same time radically alters his personality. Are such actions justified despite their unfortunate effects?

The casuistic principle of two-fold effect provides a formula for the solution of problems of this type. The formula is expressed in the following conditions which must be fulfilled in order for an action, which has both good and bad effects, to be regarded as morally good: (1) the action itself must not be intrinsically bad; (2) the good effect must not be a direct consequence of the bad effect; (3) the good effect must be 'directly intended': the bad effect only 'indirectly intended', or 'tolerated'; (4) the good effect must be equal to or greater than the bad effect. The operation of these conditions can be demonstrated by applying them to two hypothetical cases:

Physician A prescribes a pain-killing drug for a dying patient, which causes some shortening of his life expectancy.

Physician B prescribes a lethal dose for a dying patient in order to put him out of pain.

The principle of two-fold effect condemns B's action but allows A's on the grounds that B's prescription caused the patient's death which then relieved the pain (condition 2 violated), whilst A's prescription *intended* the good effect of alleviating pain and merely *tolerated* the bad effect of shortening life.

A second set of hypothetical cases may further clarify the way the principle is applied:

Surgeon A operates to remove a Fallopian tube in which a fetus has become implanted in order to prevent the death of the mother, thereby also destroying the fetus.

Surgeon B terminates the pregnancy of a patient whose medical condition is such that continuation of the pregnancy may kill her.

According to the operation of the principle, surgeon A acts rightly but surgeon B acts wrongly. Surgeon A has operated with the intention of removing a diseased organ, merely tolerating as an unfortunate effect the death of the fetus. Surgeon B has operated to destroy the fetus in order to save the mother's life—the end (saving life) can never justify the means (destroying the fetus). Surgeon B's action is wrong either because the operation of abortion is itself intrinsically bad (violates condition 1), or because the good effect came from the bad effect (violates condition 2), or because he intended the death of the fetus (violates condition 3).

It should be noticed that in order to put this principle into operation an 'atomistic' approach to human action has to be taken, that is to say the situation of moral decision has to be split into separate parts, consisting of the 'action itself' and the 'effects of the action'. Each part thus analysed out is then assigned a moral qualifier of 'good', 'bad' or 'indifferent'. Quite a different conclusion is obtained if we treat the action in a *unitary* manner, viewing it as an indivisible 'flow' from intention through action to predicted consequence. From such a viewpoint both surgeon A's and surgeon B's actions could accurately be described as surgical interventions designed to save the patient's life, which necessarily entailed the destruction of the fetus. Similarly both physician A's and physician B's prescriptions could be described as the introduction of substances into the patient's body designed to bring relief from pain even at the cost of life of the patient. So far as intention is concerned, all four doctors could fairly be described to be intending the best interests of the patient under their care : none of the four was intending to destroy life simply for the sake of destroying it.

Does such a unitary description of the actions of the four doctors gloss over some vital distinctions in the moral quality of their action? Exponents of the principle of two-fold effect would argue that it does, pointing out that what is missing is a distinction between *direct attack* on human life or fetal life, and actions which may *indirectly* cause death or fail to prevent death. Physician B and surgeon B, they would argue, deliberately destroyed life. Such direct taking of human life is in a class apart, not excusable by references to intentions to benefit the patient.

In order to explore this argument further it becomes essential to examine the distinction between causing death directly and causing death indirectly. The first thing that is necessary, is to abandon the use of the word 'attack' in this context. Like the use of the word 'murder' discussed earlier in the chapter, this usage carries misleading and unjustified overtones of malicious or hostile intent, the *desire* to hurt, to cause injury. Surgeon B has no more a hostile intent towards the fetus than does surgeon A. Both surgeons, we may safely assume, would prefer that the pregnancy should continue, did the patient's condition allow it. Nor is the physician who knows his injection will kill the patient an 'attacker'. His action is designed to prevent further suffering not cause it. In reality the only distinction which remains between the actions is the directness or indirectness of the lethal effects of the steps taken. In the case of the administration of high dosages of pain-killers or removal of organs containing fetuses, death is at one stage removed, as it were. Nevertheless, death is still a consequence of the action, which *the agent foresees*. When this is realised, the distinction between direct and indirect causation of death becomes somewhat tenuous. In no case can the consequent death be described as accidental or unintentional, since, whether direct or indirect, it is a consequence of the action of which the agent is aware before deciding to carry it out. In such a situation it seems less than honest to say that the death was 'tolerated' but not 'intended'. The point is that, however much the agent might have preferred to avoid it, it is a result of his action which he foresaw, and therefore for which he is responsible.

On these grounds it seems that the principle of two-fold effect introduces distinctions which obscure rather than clarify the relationship between the general moral principle of respect for life and the particular situations of clinical dilemma in which its application is in doubt. The outcome of such a criticism is not that there are no moral objections to administering lethal drugs to patients (several objections will be discussed in Chapter Six), but merely that arguments against such an action are not helpfully sustained by this kind of application of the means-ends distinction. Different kinds of argument are needed to clarify the doubts and difficulties which surround medical decisions about life and death. What needs to be further explored is not the abstractions of the intrinsically good or intrinsically bad action (as though there could be such a thing as actions in themselves distinct from the agents who carry them out), but rather the nature of the relationship between the doctor and the patient and the way in which this relationship is defined and controlled by the obligation to seek the patient's welfare.

Thus the conclusion of our examination of the use of the means-ends category is that it has potential value as a way of defining the limits and requirements of relationships between persons, but that its use to split up intention, action and consequence in the moral decisions of individuals distorts and clouds the real issues. As a general comment on our (admittedly) brief survey of the operation of casuistic principles, we may say that the assumptions upon which such an endeavour is based appear to miss a vital point. Casuistry sets about the deductive application of moral rules to particular situations through the use of formal principles of argument. What is missing in such an approach is any consideration of the persons who hold the principles and the persons to whose circumstances the principles are applied. A rule-governed approach to morality becomes, by the logic of its position, a wholly depersonalised one. The point is succinctly made by a modern Catholic theologian:

'What alone is morally decisive ... is the total sense of an action as seen in the concrete situation to which it is a response, and as judged in the light of man's fundamental vocation as a person' (Johann, 1968, p. 34).

## Summary

We have examined in this chapter two attempts to base ethics on universal principles: the Kantian formulation in terms of categorical imperatives; and the theory of natural law, which is based ultimately on a conception of divine eternal law. Although the notion of the universalisability of moral obligations has been seen to be an important formal requirement for a consistent moral viewpoint, many difficulties have been found in the attempt to construct a set of universally applicable moral laws. Elements of religious commitment have been identified as essential components of systems of natural law, and to this extent they have been shown to be partly beyond the scope of rational analysis. Moreover, the methods of relating general moral rules to specific situations through the use of casuistic principles have been found to entail a fresh set of assumptions as well as the importation of conceptually inadequate distinctions.

On the whole, the moral law approach seems to raise more difficulties than it solves. The concept of law, by virtue of its abstract and formalised character, by-passes the personal centre of moral action. Yet paradoxically it is within this tradition that the concept of person has found its fullest articulation. It remains to be seen in the next chapter whether the ideal of *respect for persons*, which originates in Kant's formulations of moral obligation, will provide a more useful way of understanding the basis of moral action than does the concept of universal law.

## REFERENCES

British Council of Churches Working Party (1966). *Sex and*

*Morality*. (A report presented to but not accepted by the British Council of Churches.) London: S.C.M. Press.

Duncan, A. R. C. (1957). *Practical Reason and Morality*. London: Nelson.

Fletcher, J. (1967). *Moral Responsibility: Situation Ethics at Work*. London: S.C.M. Press.

Flood, P. (1969). *Abortion: Commentary on the Abortion Act 1967*. London: The Catholic Truth Society.

Hayes, E. J., Hayes, P. J. & Kelly, E. (1964). *Moral Principles of Nursing*. New York: Macmillan.

Heron, A. (ed.) (1963). *Towards a Quaker View of Sex: An essay by a group of Friends*. London: Friends Home Service Committee.

Johann, R. O. (1968). Love and Justice. In *Ethics and Society*. Ed. De George, R. T. London: Macmillan.

Kant, I. (1785). *Fundamental Principles of the Metaphysics of Morals*. Translated by T. K. Abbott (Library of Liberal Arts Edition 1949). New York: Bobbs-Merrill.

Marshall, J. (1960). *The Ethics of Medical Practice*. London: Darton Longman and Todd.

Pappworth, M. H. (1967). *Human Guinea Pigs: Experimentation on Man*. London: Routledge and Kegan Paul.

Pius XII (1957). Allocution to Doctors and Students, *Acta Apostolicae Sedis*, Vol. XXXXIX, n. 17-18.

Rogers, C. R. (1961). *On Becoming a Person*. Boston: Houghton Mifflin.

Smith, H. L. (1970). *Ethics and the New Medicine*. Nashville: Abingdon.

St. John-Stevas, N. (1971). *The Agonising Choice: Birth Control, Religion and the Law*. London: Eyre and Spottiswoode.

Symmers, W. St. C. (1968). Not Allowed to Die. *British Medical Journal*, **1**, 442.

Vann, G. (1965). *Moral Dilemmas*. London: Collins.

Waddington, C. H. (1942). *Science and Ethics*. London: Allen and Unwin.

Welty, E. (1960). *A Handbook of Christian Social Ethics I*. London: Nelson.

# CHAPTER FIVE

# Respect for Persons

'May I never see in the patient anything else but a fellow creature in pain.' These words from the prayer of the physician Maimonides express an ideal toward which all medical intervention in the life of another person is directed. The philosophy which gives theoretical backing to this statement of moral commitment is the view which makes respect for persons a normative concept in ethics. As we have already noted (Chapter Four), this concept finds its origin in Kant's assertion that moral agents are of supreme value, because they are capable of rational choice.

We shall now explore the full implications of this approach by looking more closely at the notions of 'person' and 'respect'. In the course of this exploration we shall have to deal with two major sources of criticism of this type of theory: Determinism, which denies the possibility of freedom in human action; and Egoism, which traces all human motivation to self-interest. The need to make a full analysis of these conflicting views means that most of this chapter will be taken up with rather abstract philosophical discussion, in preparation for a full exploration of the practical problems of medical ethics.

## Person

The term 'person' functions as a description of the *status* which we grant to human beings over against other animals and inanimate objects. Personal being is held to be of particular character which demands special consideration. The nature of this status is conveyed in the famous words of the American Declaration of Independence: 'We hold these truths to be self-evident, that all men are created equal, that they are endowed by their Creator with certain inaliénable rights, that among these are Life, Liberty and the pursuit of Happiness'. Problems arise, however, in the precise definition of the personhood to which these rights belong, and in the nature of the respect which such rights demand. We shall now examine each of the critical terms in more detail.

## WHAT IS A PERSON?

Kant approached the definition of person through the concept of reason. In his view a person was a rational being, that is a being capable of reasoning from particular situations to general rules and of applying these rules consistently to himself and others. A precondition for doing this was the freedom to choose between alternatives. The difficulty of this kind of definition for some of the dilemmas of medical practice is that many individuals who possess sentient, human life would not fulfill these conditions, as the following example illustrates:

A severely mentally subnormal girl, aged fourteen, was admitted to a general hospital for an operation. Her head and body were grossly enlarged, her arms and legs exceptionally small. She had a very low level of intelligence, and animal grunts were a substitute for speech. Her parents were closely attached to the girl. In particular, the mother arranged the life of herself and her husband entirely round her needs. (Holidays had been sacrificed because the mother refused to leave the child's side, and the father had relinquished a good job in another part of the country so that his daughter could be admitted to this particular hospital.)

The operation for which the child was admitted was successful, but she later developed a chest infection which brought her very close to death. She was placed in an oxygen tent, put on a course of antibiotics and 'specialed' by a team of nurses. Why were such efforts made? Would it have been better to allow her to die peacefully, thus relieving her parents of their abnormal life (although a life they seemed to want)?

Since this patient was not capable of rational and free choice, why was her life respected by the hospital staff? Why were they not entitled to regard her as a badly damaged animal, whose life should not be prolonged unnecessarily? There must, it seems, be some important considerations apart from rationality which ensure that the subnormal are accorded the same rights as other patients. If we can discover what these considerations are, we may get to a more adequate definition of person than the purely rationalist one.

Could we regard 'reverence for life' (*see* Schweitzer, 1970) as the prevailing value which prevents arbitrary killing of the subnormal human being? This concept may give some insight into the hesitation which would be felt in destroying any sentient being for reasons of convenience, but such a broad notion of sanctity of life is not universally respected. There are many instances in medical practice in which biological existence is terminated, on the grounds that *human* life is not at stake. The following case provides an example of this:

A patient was found to have an anencephalic fetus. She was admitted to hospital for induction of labour. The surgeon from the liver transplantation team came to see both parents to ask for permission to use the liver as soon as the baby was born. Consent was obtained although the parents were very distressed. The nursing staff felt that it was contrary to the usual approach to a woman facing labour to seek consent in these circumstances and that it aggravated an already tragic situation. The child was kept alive on a respirator until the liver could be removed.

This example raises problems about the rightness or wrongness of treatment of the mother, but not of treatment of the anencephalic fetus. In its case there seems little doubt that a borderline had been crossed allowing it to be considered as a liver donor, even although its biological existence could be maintained by mechanical means. Such a human-like creature, being devoid of a brain, could not be regarded as a person. The difference is not one of capacity for independent existence only (haemodialysis patients are in this category), but of the type of relationship with other human beings which is possible. There never could be for the anencephalic fetus any sort of personal relationship with its parents or with any other human beings. For the severely subnormal patient some possibilities of relating remain, although they are very limited in scope.

What we are considering then in ascribing the status, person, to a living organism with humanoid characteristics is its *capacity to communicate and be communicated with*, both at a rational and at an emotional level. It is this possibility of relationship, rather than any biological criteria alone, that determine the decision.

## THE MEANING OF 'RESPECT'

In several recent expositions of the term respect by moral philosophers the Greek term *agape*, which is normally translated as 'love' or 'charity' has been used (*see* Harris, 1968; Downie and Telfer, 1969). The term implies a combination of rational and emotional elements: the feeling of fellow humanity applied consistently and without personal bias. The theologian Paul Tillich has argued for this kind of interdependence of reason and emotion in an essay on the fundamental aspects of morality:

'Justice is taken into love if the acknowledgement of the other person as person is not detached but involved. In this way, love becomes the ultimate moral principle, including justice and transcending it at the same time' (Tillich, 1963, p. 39).

Respect, then, implies a relationship of involvement with other persons, such that our choices and intentions are governed by their aims and aspirations as well as our own. To acknowledge another person is to acknowledge the possibility of other centres of choice and intention by which our personal aspirations may be modified. It sets in the centre of morality the language of 'we' rather than the language of 'I' and 'they'.

But is it really possible to have a disinterested concern for the welfare of others? And are human beings *ever* free to make independent moral choices? These are critical questions which any defender of a respect for persons theory must answer.

## Freedom of Choice

A central feature of respect for persons theory is its stress on the possibility of free choice open to persons. Yet one can easily think of examples of medical intervention in which the patient's *inability* to make choices for himself is assumed. This is the whole basis of psychiatric certification and the exercise of protective custody over a patient.

A calculated risk is taken when it is decided to relax supervision in the case of patients with suicidal or self-mutilation tendencies. At one hospital in which I worked as a charge nurse the routine was to keep regular contact with such patients even after discharge. In one case a patient failed to turn up for a follow-up clinic appointment. Normally a call by the mental welfare officer would be made in such cases, an appointment being made for the following week. However, in this instance it was decided to leave the patient for two weeks and then recall him to the out-patient clinic. When this appointment notification was sent out the patient's father replied informing the hospital that the patient had killed himself the previous week.

In such a case the hospital staff might have blamed themselves for failing in their duty to limit the patient's freedom for his own self-protection. Such an exercise of control over other people is justified on the grounds that they are incapable of deciding for themselves what is best for them. The hospital authorities exercise judgment on their behalf in the same way that parents take decisions on the behalf of young children. But problems arise about the limits of such an exercise of control over another person's life:

A young patient with a severe psychiatric illness, into which she had some insight, saw herself as getting older with no prospects of ever getting married and having a family. It was beneficial to her condition that she should be encouraged to mix and participate in social activities as much as possible. She had quite a large personal income, and, with her thoughts turning towards marriage, she seemed likely to fall prey to some psychopathic fortune hunter who might make her pregnant and then persuade her into marriage. It was therefore decided to add a contraceptive pill to her medication. Since she was a Roman Catholic and would have objected to such a measure, this was done without her knowledge. The decision was taken after full discussion between the medical and nursing staff, on the grounds that the patient was so incapacitated by her illness as to be incapable of controlling her own actions according to the standards of sexual morality she would normally respect.

The justification of the administration of a contraceptive pill to this patient, against her known wishes, would be that because of her illness she lacked responsibility for her own actions. Yet is such an encroachment on another person's liberty justified? In this case the notion of acting for the benefit of the patient may begin to look like taking over total control of another person's life. In order to explore this point further we need to look more closely at assumptions about 'being responsible' and 'lacking responsibility'.

## RESPONSIBILITY

To consider a person responsible for his actions is in a literal sense to hold him answerable for them. We expect him to be able to give reasons for the actions he took; and we assume that he could have acted otherwise than he did, and that therefore it is appropriate to praise him or blame him for those actions he did decide upon. However, the meaning of the innocuous looking phrase 'could have acted otherwise' is by no means easy to pin down. How do we know that a person could have acted other than he did? The clearest way of establishing this is to identify cases in which a person is clearly *not* free to act otherwise, and therefore not answerable for his actions. Two such conditions are usually identified: (1) Unavoidable ignorance; and (2) compulsion.

### Unavoidable Ignorance

The first condition exempts individuals from responsibility

when they could not have been expected to know what consequences would follow from their actions in a given situation. Very young children and persons whose intelligence has never developed beyond a very early stage are incapable of reasoning from action to consequence except in the simplest of situations. Actions carried out by adults of normal intelligence fall into this category when they are clearly accidental and not the result of avoidable negligence. (A nurse giving medicine from a bottle incorrectly labelled by the manufacturer would not be responsible for adverse consequences, but failure to check an unlabelled bottle would carry responsibility.) The extent to which ignorance of consequences is avoidable is not an open-and-shut matter. Frequently it is a matter of degree, and partial or diminished responsibility may be the most accurate description of the person's answerability.

The definition of ignorance becomes more difficult in the case of mental illness. The M'Naghten ruling (based on a trial for murder in 1843) exempts a person from responsibility, if it can be proved that he 'was labouring under such a defect of reason from disease of the mind as not to know the nature and quality of the act he was doing or if he did know it that he did not know he was doing what was wrong'. This approach to a definition of lack of responsibility due to mental illness has been much criticised by experts in forensic psychiatry. (For a survey of the criticisms see Overholser, 1959.) A major criticism is that it allows no grounds for exemption from responsibility of persons who know what they are doing, but are unable to prevent themselves from doing it. This point brings us to the second, and much more complex, condition for exemption from responsibility—that of *compulsion*.

## Compulsion

As with the first condition, it is easy to identify obvious examples of compulsion exempting from responsibility. When a person's actions are caused or prevented by external forces which he cannot overcome, we do not consider him to be free to act otherwise. (In an emergency situation, a doctor is not responsible for the deaths of people he cannot reach in time.) Other people may compel a person to act in a certain way through the use of hypnosis, drugs, or threats of physical violence, and in such cases compulsion is clearly present. The matter becomes more involved if we begin to consider the possibility of *internal* compulsion. The person who compulsively steals items because of some emotional disturbance (kleptomania) is not a thief in the normal sense of the term. But if the kleptomaniac is not responsible, what about the mother who injures her children when under psychological stress (the 'battered baby syndrome')? Could she 'not have acted otherwise'? Similar questions arise concerning the socially inadequate, apparently unable to cope with the simplest practical problem, and the juvenile delinquent, whose anti-social behaviour can be seen as a product of his own internal conflicts. Eventually one begins to wonder whether *everyone*'s behaviour might be explained according to internal compulsion of one kind or another.

This conclusion leads us into a major philosophical controversy—the debate about free will and determinism. The determinists argue that *all* human action can eventually be traced to either external or internal causes. In this sense every action is compelled and it is not possible to say that the agent could have acted otherwise. The free-will theorist on the other hand, believes that an area of free choice does remain, despite the influence exerted on individuals by physical, sociological and psychological factors.


## DETERMINISM

The most thoroughgoing form of determinism was given in the philosophy of **Baruch Spinoza** (1632–77). We shall concentrate on his ideas in exposition of the determinist position. This will mean, however, that some very obscure arguments have to be expounded. Spinoza's writing provides a prime example of what is known as metaphysics— a type of philosophical theory which tries to give an overarching explanation of everything that is.

It would not be accurate to say that Spinoza *proves* that there is no such thing as freedom of choice. It is rather in the nature of an assumption from which he proceeds in order to give a coherent explanation of the universe. His basic approach can be summed up in the term *monistic*. This term implies the belief that everything that happens coheres within a unitary interdependent system. Thus human action is seen by Spinoza as not in any ultimate sense separable from the total pattern of events which constitutes nature as a whole. Every event in nature, including human action, is a function of the entire system, and the way it occurs is totally predetermined by the prior chain of causes. On this analysis interaction between persons is not different in kind from interaction between things. Both are simply sets of events in a totally inevitable succession of happenings.

A number of problems immediately present themselves to this kind of philosophical approach. The main ones are: (1) *Individuality:* How is the apparent separateness of things from another to be explained? (2) *Consciousness:* Why is it that ideas present to consciousness appear to have an independence from the world of things? (3) *Freedom:* If all events are inevitable, why is it that conscious beings think that they are free to choose between alternatives? By giving answers to these questions we shall be sketching an outline of Spinoza's philosophical system as it impinges on the debate about determinism.

## Individuality

As regards individuality, Spinoza is concerned to provide an explanation which will not break up the overall unity of nature. He argues that the totality of events is an exceedingly complex set of sub-systems of interrelationships, each part of the totality maintaining an internal unity and balance over against every other part. This tendency for parts of the system to maintain individuality in opposition to forces tending to absorb the individual into a larger unit Spinoza names *conatus* ('striving'). Diversity in nature is the result of the *conatus* of each individual part. Such individuality, however, is only a relative matter. There is no ultimate independence for any individual within the system, for, each individuality is always also contained within a more complex unity. In the last analysis there is only *one* individual—the system as a whole. (Spinoza's name for this ultimate totality is *Deus sivi Natura*—'God or Nature'.)

Nevertheless, variations in complexity are evident between different parts of the total system. A human being is a much more complex integrated unity of parts than is, say, a speck of dust. The more complex the individual part the more it is likely to maintain a relative independence of other parts. Therefore human beings appear to have autonomy, compared with objects in the inorganic world. But a greater degree of individuality does not in any way exempt human action from the chain of causes. All that can be said is that it is the product of a more complex series of interactions, and maintains a greater degree of stability and constancy in the face of changing external conditions. Such autonomy is always relative only, never absolute.

## Consciousness

A natural reaction to this kind of description of human individuality is to object that Spinoza has omitted the vital factor of consciousness, which seems to set human life in a class apart from other forms of individuality in nature. It seems obvious that human beings do not differ *only* in complexity of internal organisation, but also in being self-aware, having knowledge of past, present and future, reflecting, reacting and planning, and so on. In reply to such an objection Spinoza would concede the uniqueness of consciousness, but *not* the independence of the world of thought from the world of physical events. The psychical, he argued, is in no sense a different world from the physical: it is simply a different aspect of the same world. Therefore every object in nature may be regarded either as a set of interrelated physical events or as a set of interrelated ideas. To speak of ideas divorced from things or of things devoid of ideas is to draw false and misleading distinctions. Every thing is also a set of ideas, even although it may not be conscious of its ideational aspect. There can be no physical event which is not also a psychical event, nor any psychical event which lacks a physical correlate. The consequence of this is that, whatever else consciousness does, it does not give independence from the chain of physical causes.

The assertion of the inseparability of the physical from

the psychical is perhaps the most difficult part of Spinoza's system. It only makes some sense when it is seen against the background of alternative ways of defining the relationship between the world of ideas and the world of things. Some philosophical systems set up an unbridgable gap between these two worlds (Dualism); other systems either reduce the world of ideas to the world of things (Materialism) or find ultimate reality only in the world of ideas (Idealism). Spinoza's philosophy avoids all three of these alternatives at the cost of (a) asserting the pervasiveness of ideas throughout the physical world (even when there is no consciousness of such ideas); and (b) denying the possibility of 'pure' thought, that is, of ideas which exist independently of the world of physical causes.

## Freedom

But why is it, then, that those individuals which are *conscious* of the world of ideas suppose themselves to possess a freedom from the physical order of cause and effect. Spinoza explains this in terms of the concept of *conatus*. Consciousness provides an awareness of the striving for individuality, and this awareness generates an illusion of freedom. An object like, say, a coffee cup has a degree of relative independence from those other objects around it. It possesses sufficient internal unity to maintain itself against a number of changes in the environment. But it does not possess that degree of complexity of internal organisation which allows for consciousness of this separateness. Human beings, on the other hand, possess some awareness of the chains of events or ideas which constitute their individuality. They are conscious of their own striving to maintain an internal unity and balance throughout environmental change. But the possession of such awareness is no gain in freedom. Certainly human beings tend to *believe* themselves to be independent beings, masters of their own fate, free to decide. However, they have merely allowed their consciousness to confuse them. Having become aware of their *conatus*, they suppose themselves to be free. In reality they have no more control over their striving for individuality than they have over the external forces which militate against it. Seen clearly and without illusion, that which is named 'I' is no more than a series of psychophysical events whose succession depends wholly on the interrelationship of internal and external forces.

The conclusion from these definitions of individuality, consciousness and freedom is that the only freedom possible for conscious beings is freedom from error or illusion. There can be no independence from the chain of cause and effect which operates throughout nature. The only truly free man is the man who discards the illusions, prejudices and self-deception which accompany the supposition of free choice, and who knows that the way he and others act is the way they inevitably act. Such a man discards all notions of pain and pleasure, praise and blame, and is concerned only with that which is possible for him—clarity of understanding.

## DEFENCES AGAINST DETERMINISM

How are we to assess a theory like Spinoza's? In many respects it seems to be in harmony with modern developments in scientific theory. His attempts to maintain a psychophysical unity of explanation, and his use of the concept of internal balance to account for individuality, anticipate by three centuries much contemporary discussion in psychology, biology and philosophy of science. In particular his assertion of universal causality seems more and more justified by the expansion of the 'sciences of man'. As psychological and sociological theories become more sophisticated, the possible area of human self-determination seems to narrow down to vanishing point. Certainly such theories are still clumsy predictors of human behaviour and the interrelationship of the different sciences which study man is as yet far from clear, but many modern thinkers feel sure that a comprehensive scientific explanation of all aspects of human behaviour is now possible in principle, even if its achievement is still many years in the future.

Most modern defenders of determinism, however, would not find it necessary to support Spinoza's whole metaphysical system in order to establish the absence of free will. A more common kind of argument is one which asserts the implausibility of the hypothesis of human freedom. How can we assert free will when we can see for ourselves that the actions of individuals vary in accordance with differences in character and environment? In any case, the argument goes on, would we not regard it as preferable for human action to be predictable, consistent, patterned, than for it to be random, unpredictable or subject to the whim of the individual?

The defender of a theory of free will against the deterministic analysis has a number of methods of defence at his disposal. Against a metaphysical system like Spinoza's he may simply elaborate an alternative system of metaphysics, one which begins with the possibility of freedom as a presupposition. Against the more modern science-based type of argument, he can press for greater clarity of definition of the terms 'free' and 'determined'. If 'determined' means no more than 'consistent and predictable' then the free will theorist need not see a threat to his point of view. He can concede that human beings do not act randomly, but rather in accordance with policies or principles. These principles, he then goes on to argue, are not forced upon individuals, but are rationally chosen by them from a range of alternatives. So long as determinism is arguing about probabilities not necessities it need not be in opposition to theories of free will. These theories can remain in force provided the possibility that the individual might have acted otherwise is left open.

Many versions of determinism, however, will not allow for this possibility. The so-called choice of principles or the possibility of acting unpredictably will, it is argued, also yield to explanation, if we know enough about all the influences acting upon the agent at the time of decision. When the whole picture is known, it will be seen that there could have been only one possible action for this person at this moment. This 'strong' form of determinism goes beyond scientific assertion (which is always in the form of probabilities) to the assertion of a belief in the total regularity of events in nature.

The debate between the advocates of determinism and the advocates of free will has the appearance of being a perennial one in philosophy. It would be rash to suppose that either side can be conclusively proved wrong. All that can be done by way of comparative assessment is to discover what consequences for ethical theory each view has. One set of consequences may then appear to be more acceptable to us than the consequences of the opposing view.

Approached in this way determinism can be seen to have some unfortunate implications for the moral theorist. In the first place it undermines the validity of rational argument. Since human beings inevitably hold the views they hold, it is pointless to look for reasons for or against any particular opinion. This consequence of the theory can be neatly turned against the deterministic philosopher's own use of argument to defend his position. As J. R. Lucas (1970, p. 115) points out:

'They want to be considered as rational agents arguing with other rational agents; they want their beliefs to be construed as beliefs, and subjected to rational assessment; and they want to secure the rational assent of those they argue with, not a brain-washed repetition of acquiescent patter. Consistent determinists should regard it as all one whether they induce conformity to their doctrines by auditory stimuli or a suitable injection of hallucinogens: but in practice they show a welcome reluctance to get out their syringes, which does equal credit to their humanity and discredit to their views.'

A second consequence of the assertion of total determinism is that it virtually empties of all intelligibility the moral concepts of 'responsibility' and 'obligation'. The problem is summarised in the phrase 'ought implies can'. It makes no sense to tell a person that he ought to do X or to hold him responsible for failing to do X, if he was bound to do it or to fail to do it. The following example illustrates the point:

A patient, aged 29, with kidney disease, requires haemodialysis regularly. He is booked in for overnight treatment three times a week but frequently fails to turn up on the correct night. His excuse is always that it was not convenient, usually because he was 'away with the boys'. (His friends have been known to sleep in their car in the hospital car park overnight.) Fortunately it is usually possible to fit him in at other times for at least one of his three treatment sessions per week. He has been warned that without the treatment he will die within a month. Should another more deserving a person be allocated his regular place?

If the patient inevitably acted in an erratic manner, there would be no point in calling him 'irresponsible' or in any way blaming him for failing to turn up for treatment. Spinoza did not hesitate to accept this as a conclusion of determinism. He considered that the rational man would free himself of the mistaken idea that people should be praised or blamed for their actions or that they should be expected to act differently from the way they had acted. Some recent exponents of determinism, however, have tried to salvage the meaning of obligation and responsibility by interpreting them as descriptions of methods of influencing behaviour. On this interpretation, saying 'you ought to do X' is an attempt by us to influence the behaviour of the person to whom the remark is directed; and holding a person 'responsible' for his actions is simply saying that he is open to influence by praise or blame. Thus calling the young man in the example 'irresponsible' is no more than a tactic used by us to try to change his behaviour. Inanimate objects or persons under the control of external forces are not held responsible, because they are not amenable to influence by persuasion. 'Obligation' and 'responsibility' are operative only when actions are at least partially the product of a person's inclinations and general character. These actions are just as much within the sway of causation as any others, but the balance of cause and effect may be altered by our approving or disapproving of them.

Is such a modified account of obligation and responsibility convincing? Perhaps we can say little more than that to those philosophers *already* convinced about determinism, it is. Other ethical theorists however prefer the puzzles posed by free will to the puzzles posed by determinism. They would defend their point of view by pointing to the different methods by which problems are tackled in ethics and in scientific theory. The scientific method is based on the search for generalisations on the basis of which predictions can be made. The method of ethics is based on the investigation of individual decision and of the lines of reasoning by which decisions are reached. Science seeks causes: ethics seeks reasons. Both may well be valid ways of viewing a situation. But they ask different questions, on the basis of different assumptions, and as a result the answers they arrive at appear to be in contradiction.

This point of view is well represented by the conclusions reached by Kant on the subject of freedom of the will. Viewed from the point of natural science, Kant conceded, freedom is an impossibility, since such a point of view presupposes that all events have a prior cause. But viewed from the point of view of the moral agent, freedom is a necessary hypothesis. Without the presupposition of freedom, the moral law is emptied of all its authority, becoming merely an external imposition upon the individual, instead of his own freely adopted principles of action. Therefore, for ethical theory freedom must be assumed, although it can never be proved.

### Self-Interest and Benevolence

Up to this point we have been arguing for the possibility of freedom of choice. This appears to be an essential component of the concept of person or moral agent. But another set of difficulties threatens the notion of *respecting persons*. We have already seen that the term respect implies an active concern or 'love' for others. Many philosophers have regarded the notion of disinterested love for others to be as illusory as the notion of free will. Their point of view would be shared by many 'plain men' who regard themselves as common sense realists about human behaviour. The following case illustrates how, even in the case of close family, the welfare of others may be disregarded:

Mr X, a widower of 70 years, resided with his only son and daughter-in-law. Normally a very active man, he had a sudden cerebral haemorrhage one day and became hemiplegic.

As his daughter-in-law was unwilling to nurse him at home, he was admitted to a geriatric ward for medical treatment and rehabilitation with a view to returning home. After several weeks in hospital this aim was achieved and he was now reasonably mobile. His relatives, however, refused to take him home, as they seemed to think they could not manage to look after him, and did not relish undertaking nursing tasks.

This refusal had a very bad psychological effect on Mr X. He now realised his whole future would be that of a patient in this ward or some other hospital ward waiting for death. He became detached, disinterested, depressed and ate very little. It seemed to the staff that the attitude of the relatives amounted to a sentence of death.

The most consistent attack on the possibility of having a disinterested concern for the welfare of others comes from the school of philosophy known as Egoism. Perhaps the most celebrated exposition of egoism in modern western philosophy is that of the English political theorist **Thomas Hobbes** (1588–1679). Many subsequent discussions of the concept of self-love—notably those of Joseph Butler and of David Hume—were written in reaction to Hobbes' views.

### SELF-INTEREST AND MORALITY

Hobbes set himself the task of analysing the structures of political, social and personal life into simple components for which precise definitions could be given, and from which a rational and comprehensive account of human behaviour could be constructed. He identified two basic elements out of which all voluntary action developed— *desires* and *aversions*. These, he said, were the imaginations of action, which themselves were the imperceptible beginnings of movement *towards* (desire) or *away from* (aversion) objects. Thus every human action aims at the satisfaction of desire, or at least at the avoidance of those things not desired. What men desire they call 'good': what they have an aversion for they call 'bad'.

However, it is not always possible for the individual to satisfy every desire. His desires may be in conflict with one another, or more commonly in conflict with the desires of other individuals. The restriction of desire therefore becomes necessary in order to ensure maximum long-term satisfaction for the individual. Men have to enter into agreements with one another about the limitation of individual satisfaction. Without such a mutual restriction of desire Hobbes believed that human societies would be in a state of perpetual violence and chaos, a state in which the life of man would be 'solitary, poor, nasty, brutish and short'.

The mutual limitations of liberty to seek what one wants for oneself Hobbes called the Laws of Nature. The first of these laws was 'that every man ought to endeavour peace, as far as he has hope of obtaining it; and when he cannot obtain it, that he may seek, and use, all helps and advantages of war'; the second law, 'that a man be willing when others are so too, as much as he shall think it necessary for peace and for the defence of himself, to lay down his right to all things; and be contented with so much liberty against other men as he would allow other men against himself'. In order for these first two laws to be put in operation individuals have to enter into relationships of mutual trust which Hobbes called covenants. The third law of nature safeguards these agreements: 'that men perform their covenants made'.

To summarise: Hobbes' theory traces all interpersonal transactions to the motive of self-interest. It is because *I* need a secure and non-exploitive society in order to satisfy *my* desires that I am prepared to safeguard the interests of others. Were such a consideration of others not to my advantage, I would not enter into the restrictive agreements of law and morality. Purely disinterested action is simply not possible, since it would involve acting in a way that was not based on satisfaction of desire.

There is in this Hobbesian description of human behaviour what might be called a bracing realism. Such an account undercuts hypocritical posturing about our supposed unselfishness. Moreover, the belief in the pervasiveness of self-interest has found a new lease of life in twentieth-century thought through Sigmund Freud's theories of human motivation (*see* Chapter Two). The person devoted to good works is now seen with a more cynical eye, especially when his charitable fervour is imbued with an attitude of patronisation. Beneath such an attachment to the problems of others the Freudian interpreter finds lurking unconscious needs for self-satisfaction.

Yet, even if we grant the dubious motivation of some people's concern for others, there are points at which the egoistic philosopher's explanations in terms of self-interest seem somewhat contrived and far-fetched. The degree of risk and of dedication associated with some aspects of medical care do not seem to have a direct bearing on any advantage, material or emotional, which the doctors and nurses stand to gain by their involvement in medicine rather than in some other profession. The dilemma expressed in the following situation could surely not arise according to Hobbes' definition of natural law. For, in such a definition, no-one would consider exposing themselves to a serious degree of risk for the sake of patients.

Staff employed in haemodialysis units run the risk of developing a form of hepatitis which can be fatal. All reasonable precautions are taken to protect the staff, but is it right to subject them to risk, particularly when many of them have young families dependent on them? Yet, without the staff, the patients, who may also have dependants, would not survive.

Another example from hospital practice, which seems to cast doubt on the self-interest theory, is to be found in the recent enquiries into maltreatment of patients in some psychiatric and mental subnormality hospitals. (HMSO, Cmnd. 3975, 4557, 4861.) Superficially these reports might appear to back up Hobbes' analysis, since they provide evidence that some individual members of the nursing profession disregard the welfare of their patients, or even actively exploit patients to their own advantage. But what emerges just as significantly from these reports is the action of those members of staff of these hospitals who saw fit to report incidents of misconduct. These reports were often made by junior staff members who had nothing to gain, and much to lose, by defending their patients' welfare in opposition to the attitudes of some of those who held power in the institution (*see*, for example, *Whittingham Hospital Report*, chapter 3; *Ely Hospital Report*, chapter 7).

In answer to such objections, the defender of the self-interest theory will reply that, even though there was an element of personal risk, the individuals referred to *must* have had *something* to gain from their actions on the patients' behalf, or they would not have done them. But such a reply indicates that the egoistic theorist is playing a logical game which he can never lose. *Whatever* evidence we bring to show that some actions are not self-interested, the exponent of egoism will automatically discard it on the grounds that somewhere a self-interested motive lurks. The logic of such a position seems to be something like this: If a person does X voluntarily, he must want to do X, therefore he is doing X to satisfy a desire, therefore his action is self-interested. The only way to defeat this approach is to show the incorrectness of the logic. The weakness in the argument is the jump from saying that a person does X because he wants to, to saying that he does X in order to gain the satisfaction of doing X. A parent may gain much satisfaction from caring for his children and watching them growing up healthily and happily, but it is an odd twist of argument to say that the parent cares for his children *in order to* gain this satisfaction. (In practice the opposite is frequently the case. The parent constantly seeking 'the rewards' of parenthood is apt to miss them.) Similarly, doctors and nurses can be presumed to get some satisfaction out of caring for the sick, but it does not follow that their only motive is the emotional and material satisfaction they can get out of the practice of medicine. What the egoist fails to establish is why love of one's children should be any less credible a motive than the gain to self-esteem which parenting may bring; or why the desire to help people recover from illness should be less credible than the self-concerned motives which lead people into the health and welfare professions. There seems to be no compelling reason for reducing all other-directed motives to self-interested ones.

## BENEVOLENCE AND MORALITY

We get interesting further commentary on the relationship between motive and action in the writing of the Scottish philosopher **David Hume** (1711–76), who shared Hobbes' desire to analyse morality in terms of human nature as we know it, but who did not find it necessary to reduce everything to self-interest. Hume, like Hobbes, had no taste for idealistic speculation about morality. He saw as his purpose the introducing of the 'experimental method of reasoning into moral subjects'. The result of his 'experimental' approach (that is, an approach based on the study of what people actually experience) was the conclusion that the decisive aspects of moral judgment were emotional rather than rational. The ability to reason, he considered, was useful only for establishing matters of fact and for tracing the relationships between ideas. It could not move us to action. To achieve this a *sentiment* of approval or disapproval was necessary.

Up to this point Hume seems to have much in common with Hobbes, but he then goes on to diverge decisively from egoism by putting the motive of benevolence on an equal footing with the motive of self-interest. He believes that simple observation establishes the fact that we approve of things beneficial to others just as much as we approve of things beneficial to ourselves. In general, it is those things which bring pleasure directly or those things which, because of their usefulness, being pleasure indirectly, that are approved of by most men. The strength of their approval is no less if the pleasure obtained is someone else's rather than their own.

Why is it that the pleasure of others gains our approval? Hume explains this in terms of the concept of *humanity*: 'One man's ambition is not another man's ambition, nor will the same object satisfy both; but the humanity of one man is the humanity of every one, and the same object touches this passion in all human creatures'. (*Enquiry into the Nature of Morals*, p. 273.) In other words, our approval of the pleasure of another is based on our ability to share in his experience as though it were our own.

Elsewhere Hume uses the notion of *sympathy* to express the same idea. Sympathy is evoked in us because of an association of feelings. We observe anger or sadness, frustration or joy in another and this observation of facts becomes infused with emotion through the association of the idea of myself with the idea of the other person. Even between total strangers such a communication of feeling is possible because human experience and human emotional expression are very similar from person to person. But, naturally, the closer the other is to me, through blood relationship or through friendship, the more will I resonate to his feelings.

Thus Hume sees no opposition between self-interest and benevolence, and no need to reduce one to the other. Anything which serves the common cause of humanity will be naturally approved by all reasonable men. There is at least one negative consequence of Hume's views, however. He has no time at all for what he calls 'the whole train of monkish virtues'—by which he means celibacy, fasting, humility and the like—even although some men may approve of them. In Hume's estimation they must be classed as vices rather than virtues, since they are neither useful nor enjoyable to anyone.

Part of the enjoyment of reading Hume's philosophy is his entertainingly polemical style. His concluding remarks on monkishness are well worth quoting for this reason alone:

'A gloomy, hare-brained enthusiast, after his death, may have a place in the calendar; but will scarcely ever be admitted, when alive, into intimacy and society, except by those who are as delirious and dismal as himself.' (*Op. cit.*, p. 270.)

There is also a more serious reason for quoting these remarks. At this point Hume has committed himself to a set of values and rejected another set. This means he has shifted from saying what men generally *do* approve of to saying what men *ought* to approve of. For, it seems plain that, however many people expressed approval of the 'monkish' virtues, Hume would still be on the side of those who prefer the amiable and useful virtues. One commentator, who is largly sympathetic to Hume's approach, has put the point as follows:

'Like so many others who have written about a fundamental, unchanging "human nature", Hume takes his notion of it largely from an examination of the thoughts, practices and sentiments of the educated and cultured eighteenth-century European.' (Kemp, 1970, p. 50.)

This leads us to the fundamental weakness of Hume's empirical approach to the problems of morality. He has explained a good deal about the origin of feelings of approval in people when they contemplate the characters and actions of themselves and others, but his theory can provide no basis for deciding whether such feelings are *appropriate*. The fact that most of Hume's contemporaries might have regarded self-denial as misguided does not tell us whether or not self-denial is morally wrong. All that it tells us is that this kind of action was disapproved of by this class of people on the basis of their general approbation of the useful and the pleasant.

The same problem arises in Hume's argument for the influence of sympathy in moral judgment. Such an emotion is entirely admirable and desirable—without it moral judgment becomes cold and inhuman. But feelings of benevolence are not adequate determinants of moral obligation. They are too prone to variation, particularity and preference. The following administrative dilemma illustrates this difficulty:

A nurse within a few years of retirement, with a long record of good service had become unreliable in attendance at the hospital, because of the need to care for an ageing mother and because of her own deteriorating health. Should she be dismissed before retirement age, thereby losing some pension and superannuation benefits, or should the hospital administration tolerate a more erratic pattern of service, thereby causing difficulties to other nurses and possibly depriving the patients of adequate nursing care at all times?

The conflict of obligation which the hospital administrator had to deal with in this case would not be assisted by Hume's analysis of sympathy through association of feeling. The administrator is perhaps more likely to feel sympathy for her colleague, identifying more easily with her than with the patients because of similarities in outlook, experience and education. Yet such a sympathetic feeling could be a very poor indicator of where the moral obligation lies. Dismissing the nurse to safeguard the welfare of the patients might well mean overriding personal feelings, and yet be the right decision.

It seems that Hume has unearthed an essential feature of moral interaction in identifying the emotional experience of sharing the feelings of others. What is lacking in his analysis, however, is an adequate treatment of the rational element in moral judgment. In Hume's theory of ethics reason is demoted to the status of a calculating machine, wholly subservient to the objectives toward which the emotions point. ('Reason', he declared, 'is, and only should be the slave of the passions.') Yet the concept of fairness, of equality of treatment irrespective of personal preference, seems as important for moral judgment as the feeling of fellow humanity, and that concept has the appearance of being a rational element. Therefore we need to explore further possibilities of an amalgamation of reason and emotion.

## Reason and Emotion

Throughout this chapter we have been testing out the ideal of respect for persons against a series of alternative viewpoints in philosophy. At no point has it been possible to prove that this ideal is a correct one, but at any rate none of the criticisms of the viewpoint has proved fatal. What we now need to establish is whether the notion of respect for persons does any more justice to the rational and emotional aspects of morality than the alternative theories do.

We can attempt to do this by elaborating the ideal of respecting persons in terms of *communication between the self and others*. The advantage of using the term 'communication' is that it does not commit us to either an exclusively rational or an exclusively non-rational analysis. Communication refers to that which links human beings together at both verbal and non-verbal levels of interaction. The singling-out of either rational or emotional elements is an abstraction from the complexity of interpersonal relationships.

Communication acknowledges the existence of another person. (We communicate with non-human animals also, but at a much less complex level.) Failure to communicate, or refusal to communicate, turns the other person into a thing, an inanimate object which can be manipulated in ways that suit us. This destruction of the personhood of others becomes very evident when, because of extensive emotional or intellectual damage, communication becomes very difficult. It is easy to see no more potentiality for senile patients than sitting around all day 'becoming cabbages' (*see Whittingham Hospital Report*, p. 6), or to feel surprise that severely mentally subnormal patients 'being so filthy dirty and animal-like in habits can appreciate such bright colours, decoration and comforts of a new building' (quoted in *Farleigh Hospital Report*, p. 13). When such an attitude predominates, damaged human beings are treated as animals or things and thereby lose all hope of personal being. At a less extreme level the threat of depersonalisation hangs over every human being, if communication with others breaks down or is badly disturbed. Many people with normal intellectual and emotional capacities experience this on being admitted to hospital. (Scottish Association for Mental Health, 1960.)

Whilst the failure of communication destroys personhood, the converse is also true: the effort to communicate and be communicated with *creates* personal being. The crucial importance of communication for the emergence of personal being can be seen in at least three ways: (1) Communication both bridges and maintains the distance between individuals. The essence of communication is its two-way character. What I communicate is responded to by another, and this response provides something *I* could not necessarily anticipate, aim at, or bring into being. Thus communication prevents me from absorbing the other into my world of needs and desires. (The totally self-centred individual is the one who never genuinely communicates with others. He is a prisoner of his own world, and he attempts to confine others in it also.) (2) Communication creates new emotional bonds, opening up possibilities of replacing prejudice and aversion with participation in what it feels like to be the other. This is what Hume was aiming at with his concept of humanity, but he limited its scope with his categories of the agreeable and the useful. The communication of emotion may be seen as a very important part of freedom, since it involves freedom from the emotional responses to which our upbringing has conditioned us in order to share emotionally in something new in the present moment of encounter with another person. (3) Communication provides the basis for consistent and controlled interaction with others, since it is a channel whereby information can be received about the effects on others of what one is doing in a situation (feedback). In theory at least, this means that our interactions need be neither random and impulsive, nor stereotyped and rule-bound, but rather a constantly self-corrective engagement with others.

Of course, all that has just been said about the personalising character of communication is only a description of what might be, not necessarily of what is. Many actual instances of human communication do not achieve the ideal of respect for persons. Communication techniques may be used to exert control over others (indoctrination, advertising); many attempts at communication re-inforce prejudice rather than destroy it; and communication may fail to provide feedback or to alter habitual ways of acting toward others. The force of our argument has merely been that, if respect for persons is a realisable ideal, then communication of a particular rational and emotional quality is a means of attaining it.

## Conclusions

A point which has emerged repeatedly in our expositions of opposing ethical theories is that all approaches rest on certain assumptions which themselves cannot be proved. This is certainly true of the approach which stresses rational and emotional communication between persons as an ideal in morality. It is, in the last analysis, making a statement of commitment, not a statement of fact. Out of such a commitment there emerge some important implications for medical ethics which can now be briefly indicated.

*Firstly*, this viewpoint places no final authority on moral rules. Since communication involves constant openness to change, the generalisations contained within rules may have to be modified in the light of a particular person's situation. *Secondly*, the values of the individual are placed above the value of benefit to the society. Of course, these two values are closely interrelated, but at least a limit is defined, namely that no amount of social benefit justifies the depersonalising of individuals. *Thirdly*, this approach sees as the surest sign of trying to benefit the other a consistent attempt to open and maintain communication with him, even in cases when personal being is only potentially present or has largely lapsed. (In the context of medical care, this does not necessarily mean discussing the patient's condition with him, but simply communicating with him in a way appropriate to his present awareness. Failure to make this attempt indicates that the patient has become simply an object to be moulded to one's own preconceptions of what is good for him.)

It is open to anyone to question that starting-point of this theory, on the grounds that its implications for medical care are unrealistic or unhelpful. Undoubtedly the use of the norm of respect for persons introduces elements of uncertainty and delay into the day-to-day decisions of morality. Treating others always as persons is costly in time and resources. In the sphere of health care it is difficult enough to develop a service which can cope with the obvious distresses of acute illness and physical injury. Trying to build in norms of personalisation also, enormously increases the complexity and cost. Moreover allowing the otherness of others makes life in societies much less secure and certain. There is always the danger (which Hobbes envisaged) of social disintegration, in which all is openness and choice and nothing can be predicted or relied upon.

The norm of respect for persons is no more exempt from criticism than the other approaches to ethics already discussed. In the last analysis it will be for the reader to decide which theoretical account of morality is the more convincing and comprehensive. Basic assumptions, as we have already observed, are not open to proof.

## REFERENCES

Downie, R. S. & Telfer, E. (1969). *Respect for Persons.* London: Allen and Unwin.

Harris, E. (1968). In *Ethics and Society*. Ed. De George. R. T. London: Macmillan.

HMSO (1969). *Report of the Committee of Enquiry into Allegations of Ill-treatment of Patients and Other Irregularities at the Ely Hospital, Cardiff.* Cmnd. 3975.

HMSO (1971). *Report of the Farleigh Hospital Committee of Enquiry*, Cmnd. 4557.

HMSO (1972). *Report of the Committee of Enquiry into Whittingham Hospital.* Cmnd. 4861.

Hume, D. (1777). *Enquiry Concerning the Principles of Morals.* Edition of Selby-Bigge, L. A., 1902. Oxford: Clarendon.

Kemp, J. (1970). *Ethical Naturalism.* London: Macmillan.

Lucas, J. R. (1970). *The Freedom of the Will.* Oxford: Clarendon.

Overholser, W. (1959). Major Principles of Forensic Psychiatry. In *American Handbook of Psychiatry II*. Ed. Arieti, S. New York: Basic Books.

Schweitzer, A. (1970). *Reverence for Life.* Translated by Fuller, R. H. London: S.P.C.K.

Scottish Association for Mental Mealth (1960). *Report of the*

*Scottish Study Group on Psychological Problems in General Hospitals.*

Tillich, P. (1963). *Morality and Beyond*. New York: Harper Row.

# CHAPTER SIX

# Some Perspectives on Current Problems

## The Relevance and Irrelevance of Ethics

The reader who has persevered to this point through expositions of four different approaches to ethics will have realised that the subject offers no simple solutions. We have seen that the following kinds of questions are discussed (with apparently unflagging enthusiasm) by moral philosophers: the relative functions of reason and emotion in moral judgment; the possibility or otherwise of freedom of decision; the relationship between self-love and benevolence; the relevance of happiness to decisions about what is morally right; the nature of moral rules and their applicability to particular situations.

The main conclusion to be drawn from our survey seems to be that every attempt to give a coherent account of the nature of morality is open to question and debate. As John Stuart Mill observed on the opening page of *Utilitarianism*:

'From the dawn of philosophy, the question concerning the *summum bonum*, or, what is the same thing, concerning the foundation of morality has been accounted the main problem in speculative thought, has occupied the most gifted intellects, and divided them into sects and schools, carrying on a vigorous warfare against one another. And after more than two thousand years the same discussions continue, philosophers are still ranged under the same contending banners, and neither thinkers nor mankind at large seems nearer to being unanimous on the subject ...'

Because of this state of perpetual debate, a person may become disenchanted with the whole activity of ethical theorising. Why bother with such tortuous argumentation, if it has no practical outcome? Yet, seen from another perspective, the lack of 'progress' in ethics may be reckoned to be its greatest advantage, since it means that every line of argument is open to constant scrutiny. A 'Final Solution' in ethical theory would presumably mean the abolition of doubt and dissent in moral discourse, since there would then be one agreed way of analysing every aspect of morality. Such a foreclosure of questioning and uncertainty would be both unhelpful and impossible to implement. At the centre of morality is the facing-up to difficult choices in new situations. The perpetual re-assessments of ethical theories mirror these complexities.

No doubt it is fortunate for doctors, nurses and especially patients, that morality is still actively pursued, whatever the lack of agreement about its theoretical foundations. In medicine, as in most other spheres of life, decisions have to be taken, routines established, attitudes taught and cultivated. The morality of medical care is a subsystem of the moral beliefs of the society within which the care is offered. Thus patients and staff already share expectations of one another's conduct and are broadly in agreement about what constitutes unconscientious or unethical behaviour.

The moral beliefs of any society, however, can be expected to have shortcomings as well as insights. When conflict arises between staff about the rightness of procedures or when public debate of medical priorities arises, the transition from morals to ethics becomes both appropriate and useful. The range of ethical theory provides alternative analyses by which each individual can assess his own convictions. Some theories will seem more reasonable and immune from criticism than others. (No doubt in this book the author's own biases and blind spots have been evident.) But perhaps the best preparation for responsible moral decision which ethics can provide is the opportunity it gives to sample theoretical analyses which, from one's own experience of morality, seem alien, unattractive even ridiculous. Ethics is rather deficient in the supply of simple answers: but when studied with an open mind it can help one to grapple with some unexpected and interesting questions.

## Current Problems

In the rest of this chapter some of these questions will be explored further by discussing how they relate to a selection of current problems in medical decision making.

Before making the selection we may briefly survey the range of problems presented in contemporary medicine. There are few areas of medical practice in which no ethical questions arise. From the very beginning of human life there are issues to be debated: Advances in genetic engineering have offered the possibilities of removal of genetic defects, pre-selection of the sex of offspring and other more radical forms of genetic manipulation (Ramsey, 1970; Hamilton, 1972). Artificial fertilisation techniques by donor insemination and by *in vitro* fertilisation and embryo transfer (Ciba Foundation, 1973) have raised both moral and legal puzzles round the question of 'natural' parentage. Improvements in genetic screening and antenatal detection of defects (Emery, 1974; Jones and Bodmer, 1974) have brought with them the dilemmas of selective abortion and of genetic counselling. The increasing incidence of medical termination of pregnancy has resulted in questioning of the meaning of the term 'therapeutic abortion'. Similarly, human death brings with it a cluster of moral problems. The question of prolongation of life sometimes arises immediately after birth, when doctors must decide whether to intervene in cases of severely deformed neonates with low survival potential (Stark, 1973). It continues with decisions about mechanical life support of the massively brain damaged, transplantating of vital organs and resuscitation of terminally ill patients. Many of these questions are crystallised in the debate about 'euthanasia' whether this term is taken to mean actively killing patients as an 'act of mercy', or desisting from over-active treatment (Dunstan, 1972).

Another range of problems concerns priorities in medical care. Although dramatic issues of birth and death capture the public imagination, equally difficult questions are implicit in the allocation of priorities in health care. This kind of problem is thrown into sharp relief by the following imaginary, but factually based, description of a situation facing a doctor in rural Africa:

We can move closer to these problems by joining a young government physician as he arrives at his first assignment. He has just finished his internship and has been assigned to serve in a rural district.

His district is 20 miles wide and 30 miles long and contains about 70,000 people. He is the only doctor. The hospital has 70 beds, and there are 110 patients. The nurse—there is only one—shows him around.

A large crowd is in the out-patient clinic, and he learns that 200 to 400 patients come each day. Two medical assistants are looking after them. The doctor will be asked to see the difficult problems. As he walks by, malnutrition, anaemia, skin problems and eye diseases are obvious ...

As they look around, the nursing sister tells him of a new patient, a woman who has been in obstructed labour for two days and now has the signs of a ruptured uterus. The operating theatre is ready if he needs it. The regional hospital with a surgeon is 140 dirt-road miles away (World Council of Churches, 1969).

In the so-called developed countries decisions about priorities are less immediately obvious. But it has become clear that simply spending more money on modern medical technology does not by itself meet the right priorities in health care. Although the U.S.A. spends 6 per cent of the Gross National Product (the highest proportion in the world) on health, it compares badly with other developed countries in mortality statistics and in general availability of routine health care. Studies of the British National Health Service reveal a more equitable distribution of medical services, but a large gap between need and treatment, especially in geriatrics, psychiatry and facilities for the mentally handicapped (Leach, 1970, chapter 11). The failure of modern medicine to bring about healthier societies and the evidence of actual damage caused by some modern treatments had led to claims that most modern health budgets cause more harm than good. In *Medical Nemesis*, Illich argues for a total reversal of present trends in health service planning:

The proliferation of medical agents is health-denying not only or primarily because of the specific functional or organic lesions produced by doctors, but because they produce dependence. And this dependence on professional intervention tends to impoverish the non-medical health-supporting and healing aspects of the social and physical environments, and tends to decrease the organic and psychological coping ability of ordinary people. (1974, p. 40f.)

Illich's warnings about the 'nemesis' of modern medicine

underline the point that the removal of specific diseases and disabilities does not of itself guarantee the enhancement of health. The identification of *diseases* and the development of effective therapies fit well into a science-based medicine, but defining norms for *health* appears much more speculative and value-laden. Yet priorities in medicine inevitably entail debates about the second kind of question. As Lambourne (1973, p. 23) points out: ' "Healthy for what?" and "Diseased from what?" are both equally important questions and provisional answers to both are always implicit in every medical act'.

Out of this wide range of problems, three will be examined in greater detail. The *abortion* debate illustrates the difficulties in defining the beginnings of human life and in establishing grounds for justified termination of pregnancy. Discussion about *care of the dying* involves analysis of assumptions about the quality of human life. *Organ transplantation* and *medical research* illustrate some of the dilemmas about priorities.

## Abortion

There is a tendency in the debate about abortion for arguments to become polarised. On the one side phrases like 'murder of the innocent' are used, whilst on the other much is made of 'the rights of women'. Yet as Roger Wertheimer has pointed out:

Few liberals really regard abortion, at least in the later stages, as a bit of elective surgery. Suppose a woman had her fifth-month fetus aborted purely out of curiosity as to what it looked like, and perhaps then had it bronzed. Who among us would not deem both her and her actions reprehensible? Or, to go from the lurid to the ludicrous, suppose a wealthy woman, a Wagner addict, got an abortion in her fourth month because she suddenly realized that she would come to term during the Bayreuth Festival. Only an exceptional liberal would not blanch at such behaviour.

Of course, in both cases one might refuse to outlaw the behaviour, but still, clearly we do not respond to these cases as we would to the removal of an appendix or a tooth. Similarly, in my experience few of even the staunchest conservatives consistently regard the fetus, at least in the earlier stages, in the same way as they do a fellow adult. When the cause of grief is a miscarriage, the object of grief is the mother; rarely does anyone feel pity or sorrow for the embryo itself. So too, it is most unusual for someone to urge the same punishment for a mother who aborts a young fetus as for one who murders her grown child (quoted in Sarvis and Redman, 1973, p. 23).

It is important, therefore, to see the nature of the arguments for and against therapeutic abortion and to determine in what sense the word 'therapeutic' is being used.

## THE STATUS OF THE FETUS

The view that protection must be given to human fetal life goes back to the early history of the practice of medicine. The Hippocratic Oath states: 'I will give no deadly drug to any, though it be asked of me, nor will I counsel such, and especially I will not aid a woman to procure an abortion'. The modern Geneva Convention Code echoes this sentiment but with a significant difference in phrasing: 'I will maintain the utmost respect for human life from the time of conception'. Even the more cautious phrasing of the latter code ascribes a certain *status* to fetal life and excludes the possibility that it may be discarded at will.

The view which regards direct abortion as morally wrong

in *all* circumstances claims that the fetus has the same right to life as that of any other individual. This point of view is most consistently presented in the official pronouncements of the Roman Catholic Church. The Papal encyclical *Casti Connubii* (1930) describes abortion as 'the direct murder of the innocent'. A handbook of Catholic social ethics elaborates this point of view by stating that the immortal soul of the individual is present from the moment of conception: 'At the moment when conception occurs in the mother's womb God infuses the soul and human life begins.... To kill this helpless creature with full knowledge and consent is to commit murder.' (Welty, 1963, p. 123.)

The association of 'ensoulment' with the moment of conception is almost universally accepted in modern Roman Catholic teaching, although it does not carry the force of dogma. Some earlier Christian teaching on the matter dated infusion of the soul rather later. Aquinas placed it at the fortieth day after conception for males (but the eightieth for females!). Augustine of Hippo and several other authorities regarded the first movement of the child in the uterus ('quickening') as a possible sign of ensoulment. Nearly all theologians, however, condemned abortion even before ensoulment on the basis of transgression of the 'natural law', forbidding interference with procreation. The modern rigorous condemnation of abortion at any point after conception is partly based on a principle of moral theology which states that if in doubt one should take no positive action. Therefore, because of the danger that a human life might be destroyed, the fetus (or more correctly the zygote-blastocyst-embryo-fetus) is to be treated at all stages as though it were a person. Some modern Protestant theologians have agreed with the Catholic absolute prohibition of abortion, though without becoming involved in the terminology of ensoulment (e.g. Bonhoeffer, 1955). A few contemporary Catholic writers have sought reformulations of the official teaching (*see* Häring, 1974), without, however, departing from the fundamental view that fetal life must be protected and respected.

To many people involved in decision-making about abortion such pronouncements may seem unnecessary, if not a little ridiculous. To them the terminology of soul, or of the will of God for each individual, may carry no meaning at all. But without feeling the need to ascribe religious values to the processes of conception and gestation, many doctors and nurses would still regard the fetus as more than merely a bundle of cells within the mother's body which can be disposed of at her request. Obviously the *viable* fetus has a status, one which is recognised in the criminal law. (In Britain, destruction of a fetus after the twenty-eighth week is a criminal offence under the Infant Life (Preservation) Act.) However, the definition of viability is only an approximation arrived at for the convenience of the formulation of law (and primarily to distinguish between still-births and miscarriages). With modern incubation techniques there is a chance of survival and normal development outside the uterus for several weeks before the twenty-eighth week. In any case, why should *viability* be regarded as the only factor relevant to respecting the status of the fetus? So far as recognisable human characteristics are concerned the progress from the basic skeletal structure and emergence of internal organs at around eight weeks to viability about twenty weeks later is a smooth and steady maturation process. No-one would confuse an aborted fetus of, say, twelve or fifteen weeks with a full term baby: but those who have to dispose of it after abortion can hardly fail to see enough similarities to make them recognise the form of a human child whose development has been violently arrested.

## THE CONCEPT OF 'THERAPEUTIC ABORTION'

At the present time laws relating to abortion vary widely from country to country. At one end of the spectrum there are countries under strong Roman Catholic influence (such as the Republic of Ireland) in which direct abortion, even to save the life of the mother, is totally prohibited. At the other end, there are some countries with very permissive legislation (e.g. Hungary, Japan) and there are some examples of the revoking of all laws relating to abortion at least in the early stages of pregnancy, leaving the matter for private decision between patient and physician controlled only by laws relating to medical care in general (the U.S.A., according to a recent Supreme Court ruling). Between these extremes there are various legislative schemes which permit abortion on therapeutic grounds. The justification for destruction of fetuses on such grounds rests on a variety of arguments: (1) The health and/or survival of the mother or of other children dependent on her are more important than the unrealised *potential* of the fetus; (2) The *expected quality* of the fetus' life is so poor that it is better for it not to experience it; (3) the *wellbeing of society* is improved by permitting abortions under certain conditions, for example when 'back street' abortion is rife, or when population policies indicate the need to lower birth rates. The word 'therapeutic' is used in very different senses in these three arguments. In the first case the patient is the mother, in the second the fetus and in the third society as a whole.

The British Abortion Act of 1967 (which applies to all

countries in the U.K. except Northern Ireland) provides an example of an attempt to give legislative expression to the first two of these arguments. The first point to be noted about this Act is that it is phrased in negative terms: it is stating the conditions under which 'a person shall not be guilty of an offence under the law relating to abortion' (Section (1), subsection (1)). Thus the context remains one of illegality of abortion, and in no sense is a *right* to receive an abortion being defined. Four conditions are then listed which allow a registered medical practitioner to perform an abortion: risk to the life of the mother; risk to the health of the mother; risk to the health of other children in the pregnant woman's family; risk of abnormality in the child. A certificate authorising the abortion must be signed by two registered medical practitioners, who are of the opinion, formed in good faith, that one of the conditions is satisfied. (In emergency cases, a special certificate requiring only one signature can be used.)

Some particular points in the phrasing of the Act should be noted: *Risk* to health must be greater if the pregnancy continued than it would be if it were terminated; In assessing *health*, 'account may be taken of the pregnant woman's actual or reasonably foreseeable environment'. (Section (1), subsection (2)); *Abnormality* (physical or mental) predicted for the child must constitute a serious handicap.

The implementation of the British legislation for the period 1968 to 1971 has been fully reported by the Lane Committee (HMSO, 1974). It documented a rise in the number of abortions on women under 45 years performed in England and Wales in the period 1969 to 1972 from 38,899 to 100,739. (This compares with a *fall* in live births in the same group from 796,528 to 724,748.) (*cit. op.*, Vol. 2, p. 17.) The most commonly used ground for abortion was risk to the mental health of the pregnant woman, mental disorder being mentioned in more than 75 per cent of cases, although psychiatrists were involved with only 6 per cent. Moreover, two thirds of those receiving abortions were unmarried, the largest number being in the 20 to 24 age group. These figures suggest that many practitioners of abortion are interpreting the 'health' clause in a wide sense, to include most situations of unwanted pregnancy. This would be presumably particularly true in the private abortion clinics, in which a high proportion of patients are young unmarried women (*cit. op.*, Vol. 2, p. 70).

It seems then that 'therapeutic abortion' can come to mean something much wider than the avoidance of physical injury or of classifiable psychiatric disorder. In the case of the British legislation at least the ambiguity of phrases like 'the pregnant woman's actual or foreseeable environment' allows virtually total discretion to the doctor. In fact, since the risks to physical health entailed by abortion in the first trimester are lower than the risks in continuing pregnancy to full term, *any* termination at this stage would appear to be sanctioned by the legislation.

## ETHICAL ISSUES

We have seen that the abortion debate contains within it two contentious areas of definition—the meaning of the phrase 'therapeutic abortion' and the sense in which 'respect for fetal life' differs from total inviolability of fetal life.

Two approaches to the morality of abortion seem to bypass the difficulties: Those forms of natural law theory which ascribe full personal status to the fetus simply refuse to accept any grounds for its destruction, even if this means that the mother's life will be lost. Conversely, some forms of social benefit theory would support abortion at the request of the mother, unless it could be clearly shown that such a practice was having an adverse effect on the majority of the population. Criticisms of both of these ethical viewpoints have already been offered at some length in previous chapters, and will therefore be repeated now only in the briefest outline.

So far as the natural law theory is concerned, it is difficult to see how the life of the fetus and the life of the mother can be regarded as on an equal footing, far less that the fetus should be given priority. As we have already observed, none of the attributes we associate with personhood—self-awareness, freedom of choice, responsibility *for* and responsibility *to* others—can yet be ascribed to the fetus. It is true, admittedly, that the newly born infant is far removed from the adult in all these respects; and, conversely, that the fetus in its later stages has some autonomy and some communication with the maternal environment. But a line (albeit a smudgy one) can be drawn at birth, because of the immediate complexification of communication and relationship which occurs. Moreover, the natural law casuistic principle which allows the indirect destruction of the fetus, when this is necessary to save the mother's life (e.g. removal of a cancerous uterus), seems to be an acknowledgment of some difference between the fetus and a living child. The same argument would not permit the destruction of the environment upon which a *living* child depends in order to save the mother.

So far as arguments for abortion in terms of social expediency are concerned, the critical question (explored at some length in Chapter Three) is how we are to define the socially beneficial. Is the welfare of society being served by allowing free choice in the matter of destruction of partially formed human life? Respect for the fetus may of course be regarded as no more than misguided sentimentality, a mere impediment to the liberty of the individual or to the economic advantage of the society. It all depends on whether regarding the fetus as just a piece of disposable maternal tissue is failing to perceive the beginnings of a separate individual. If in some sense the fetus has human individuality, then total disregard for it does not serve human values.

A modified form of Utilitarianism ('rule-utilitarianism') might try to steer a middle course between these two views. It would argue that a relatively 'liberal' law, with controls against abuse, may reach some kind of compromise between the interests of all the parties concerned. It prevents the casual destruction of fetal life, but at the same time places most weight on the prediction of consequences for either mother or child of continuing the pregnancy.

Such an approach is vulnerable to all theoretical and practical objections which are raised against utilitarian ethics. The *practical* objections concern the difficulty of predicting adverse consequences. In the majority of cases the doctor will be presented with a complex set of psychological and social variables for assessment. Unless he takes a strictly 'medical' interpretation of 'risk to health', and accepts applications only from the physically ill or from people with clearly diagnosed psychiatric disorder, he will be left with the problem of deciding how to assess the 'risks' to his patient. In the nature of the case this can never be a simple matter. The pregnant woman may herself be requesting the abortion, or she may be being pressured by parents or by the father of the child. Even if she is sure that she does not want to continue the pregnancy at the time of application, she may subsequently feel deep regret about an abortion. Assessment of the pregnant woman's feelings is made even more difficult by the need for speed of decision. Ideally she should have the opportunity to talk it over on several occasions and explore the other options open to her, but since pregnancies are often not diagnosed until the end of the second month or later and since the risks of termination escalate from the third month onwards, such time to consider is rarely available.

Estimation of what will happen to the family of the 'unwanted' child is no easier in many cases. Obviously there may be straightforward economic factors to assess, but these again will often have to be seen in the context of the predicted attitudes to the new baby of the parent or parents. Perhaps most difficult of all to decide is the degree of disruption of the present life style or future plans of the pregnant woman which can or should be tolerated. (Are disruption of an academic career, the necessity to give up a job, or the anticipated social disgrace of an illegitimate birth, undue risks to mental health?) A final consideration is the future well-being of the fetus if it is born into a situation in which the mother cannot, or will not, care for it. If a child is 'unwanted', is it better to prevent it from developing human awareness rather than subject it to the pain of rejection or the potential emotional insecurity of adoption?

The convergence of some or all these factors makes decisions about 'greatest happiness' highly subject to uncertainty.

The *theoretical* objection to the utilitarian approach concerns its assumption that actions which succeed in maximising happiness and minimising unhappiness are the same as right actions. Even if the predictions about greatest happiness could be accurate, some theorists would object to a law which sanctions destruction of a potential human life for reasons of convenience or utility, arguing that laws should not undermine the basic moral value of the sanctity of life. This objection represents a watershed in basic ethical assumptions. For one viewpoint or the other conscientious objection to the prevailing legislation is all that remains. As the Lane Committee observed:

To have to balance the life of the fetus against the health and well-being of the mother and of her existing children presents both patient and doctor with a dilemma which challenges in a most acute and often agonising form the individual consciences of both. An individual decision it must however remain: as a Committee we can only acknowledge its significance for the moral life of the individual and of society, and seek to ensure in our recommendations that such decisions are made with all the deliberation, care and earnestness they merit (1974, para 606).

Perhaps this return to the decision of the individual conscience is an unsatisfactory point at which to leave the debate. We have already seen in Chapter 2 how variable and uncertain a criterion conscience can be. Yet this seems to be the limit of ethical analysis of this issue. There comes a point where the personhood of the fetus is either an article of faith or it is not.


## The Dying Patient


When a patient dies, a natural reaction must be that medical science has failed. Such a feeling is of course irrational, since we are all aware that death comes to everyone sooner or later and that medicine has no key to everlasting life. But the focus of attention in modern medicine has been on the postponement of death through prevention and eradication of disease and the development of impressive life-saving techniques. This death-defying feature of medical technology contrasts sharply with the medical practice of earlier ages, when the doctor, like the priest, was more often than not the herald of death. Moreover, since death is no longer a common feature of life in families it exercises a curious fascination on people. Their expectations of doctors and nurses become unrealistic and their fears are crystallised in denial, evasion and anger. It is not surprising that medical personnel share some of these contemporary attitudes and find themselves both unwilling and ill-equipped to become helpers of the dying as well as 'saviours' of the living.

Many of the moral problems raised about care of the dying patient are related to these attitudes. This is almost entirely so in the case of communication with the dying patient. It is also relevant to the debate about allowing patients to die. But when arguments about actively killing patients are introduced, a fresh set of moral questions arise, as we shall see as we briefly survey each of these topic areas.

### DISCUSSING DEATH

Although it presents a great many practical difficulties and may be distressing to staff and relatives, the question of discussing death with patients does not appear to be an insoluble moral issue. It is generally accepted that we have no right to impose our attitudes on others in matters which concern them personally. (We may try to *encourage* them to take certain attitudes, but if we force these attitudes upon them we defeat our objective.) This principle of the privacy of attitudes seems to be of particular importance at the time of dying. We might say that people should be allowed to die their own deaths (so far as they are able to), not have other people's conception of a good attitude to death imposed upon them.

If this general guide-line is correct, then there can be

no absolute rules about what should or should not be said to dying patients. Hinton (1967, Chap. 10) points out that people vary so widely in their attitudes, expectations and likely reactions that the question, 'Should the doctor tell?', can have no universally accepted answer. The same conclusion is reached by many other writers. For example Saunders (*The Care of the Dying*, p. 9) has this to say:

'It is not right in principle to set out deliberately to deceive and truth must not be lighly disposed of in any situation. I do not, however, think it is essential for every patient to know he is dying and the most important principle is love, which is not sentimentality but compassion and understanding.'

Such a point of view rules out deliberate and persistent deception of patients, carried out in the interests of a policy of never telling. Wilson (1971) quotes the case of a woman suffering from inoperable cancer who was told after an exploratory operation that her gall bladder had been removed. She was not convinced by this explanation and when she persisted in questions the ward sister brought a bottle containing gall stones (not the patient's own), with the question: 'Now are you satisfied?' In such a case, communication with the patient had been totally devalued. Even in the event of the deception being successful, 're-assurance' of the patient was achieved at the cost of undermining the trust which patients place in hospital staff. Moreover, as Trowell (1971, p. 66) points out: 'It is not edifying to so many relatives to see the doctor deliberately deceiving the patient: one day a relative may himself become a patient'.

Clearly then, decisions about what should be discussed with patients need to be based on a correct assessment of what is genuinely to his benefit. Since the hearing of bad news may bring depression and the loss of the 'will to live' many physicians are hesitant to disclose a diagnosis, even in cases where there is little doubt as regards the serious-ness of the condition. This is particularly true of the diag-nosis of cancer, since in most people's mind such news is seen (often inaccurately) as the equivalent of a death sen-tence. Research carried out in a Swedish hospital, with 101 patients who were suffering from inoperable cancer (Gerle *et al.*, 1960), provides some data relevant to this issue. This study compared the reactions of those who were told the diagnosis with those who were not, and reached the conclusion:

'There are a small number of patients for whom telling the truth would be an act of needless cruelty. On the other hand, the large number of positive reactions shows that the impact need by no means be an overwhelming shock, and that it may even be of positive value to the patient during the further course of the disease.'

The authors of this study go on to emphasise the need for adequate personal counselling of patients in these circum-stances. The recent study by Kübler-Ross (1969) of 200 dying patients in a Chicago hospital has underlined both of these findings. Kübler-Ross demonstrated that nearly all dying patients come to realise what is happening, even when efforts are made to conceal information, and that, given adequate assistance, the denial, depression and anger with which the realisation was met, could give way to hope and acceptance (*see also* Kelly and Friesen, 1950).

These pointers indicate the conclusion that discussing death is at root a problem related to interpersonal com-munication within a hospital ward. The solutions to the problem are practical ones: training of nurses and doctors in sensitive communication with the dying and the pro-vision of adequate facilities and sufficient staff for the kind of service needed. To call these solutions 'practical' does not imply that they are easy to put into effect. Within the competing priorities of medicine, care of the dying may not rank very high. It depends to a large extent on the way in which the society which provides the medical care understands the health of individuals.

## PERMITTING DEATH

Just as prevalent as the fear of death is the fear of dying. Most people want to die quickly or in their sleep, fearing pain, discomfort or indignity in death (Hinton, 1967, Chap. 2). Modern methods of pain control and relief of respiratory distress have taken much away from the fantasied 'death agonies': but at the same time, new developments in control of infection and of mechanical life support create the possibility that the process of dying may be needlessly prolonged.

In discussions of what is morally permissible in the treatment of the dying there has been much juggling with Greek words: The term 'euthanasia' literally means a 'good' or 'easy' death, but in modern times it is normally used to imply 'putting people to death', either at their request or without consulting them. In view of this usage, other words have been coined: orthothanasia (Weber, 1969) and antidysthanasia (Fletcher, 1967) have been used to refer to the avoidance of a painful, prolonged or undignified death. More simply, the avoidance of a bad death may be referred to as *passive* or *negative*, euthanasia: as opposed to the *active*, or *positive*, form which involves directly causing death. We shall consider the passive forms of permitting death first, and then discuss whether they can be distinguished from active 'mercy killing'.

At least three situations raise questions about the unnecessary prolongation of life: (1) Emergency resuscitation after cardiac arrest; (2) The treatment of pulmonary infections in patients with painful terminal illness or extensive brain damage; (3) The continuation of artificial life support for patients with extensive brain damage. A fourth situation leads on to the question of active euthanasia: the treatment of severe pain in terminal illness with drugs which may shorten life.

## Resuscitation

The techniques of restarting the heart through external manual compression, electrical stimulation, or manual massage after surgical exposure all presuppose speed of decision to take action, since failure to restore circulation to the brain cells within a few minutes results in irreparable cerebral damage. For this reason alone, attempts to resuscitate may have to be abandoned if the heart is not quickly restarted, or may never be embarked upon, if it is known that there has been a considerable time lag since cardiac arrest. Because of this essential need for speed, decisions may be taken which are subsequently regretted in view of the severely brain-damaged condition which results.

A still more difficult decision is the one *not* to resuscitate certain patients, however soon attempts can be begun. This is the point at which permitting death is being suggested. In discussing this question within the context of Greatest Happiness Theory (*see* Chapter Three, p. 70), two requirements for reaching agreed policies on resuscitation were noted: (1) Decisions of this kind have to be taken in advance, since the actual situation leaves no time for deliberation; (2) Decisions have to be taken about each patient individually, not in accordance with some broad generalisation about age or medical condition. The decision in individual cases will depend on whether to restore heart beat is merely to restore irremediable suffering. The criterion is the benefit of the patient, allowing the word 'benefit' to mean more than the prolongation of life, in whatever form.

## Withholding Treatment

Pneumonia has often been described as 'the sick man's friend'. It can bring a relatively peaceful death to patients with incurable and painful diseases. The range of antibiotics now available makes it likely that such infections can be kept at bay, but should treatment of this kind be instituted, if there is no prospect of recovery for that patient? As one geriatric physician has pointed out (Agate, 1972), it may be just as blameworthy to treat pneumonia in cases in which nothing but misery will be perpetuated, as it is to fail to treat it just because a patient is elderly. Decisions have to be taken on the basis of the physician's knowledge of the individual patient, and they are rarely easily taken.

Similar questions are raised regarding patients who are brain-damaged to such an extent that there appears to be no likelihood of recovery of consciousness, far less any kind of communicative human life. In an essay discussing euthanasia Fletcher (1967) describes the case of a 20-year-old man who had been in a coma for four years: 'An auto crash hopelessly shattered his cerebral cortex. Since then only the brain stem has sustained life. All thought and feeling have been erased, and he hasn't moved a single muscle of his body since the accident.... His mother says, "My son is dead!"' If such patients develop pulmonary infections, should every effort be made to cure them?

Decisions to withhold treatment appear at first sight

to be denials of the duty of the doctor to *preserve* life, but the issue to be discussed is whether they could fulfil his commitment to *respect* it.

## Switching Off Machines

A third example of permitting death is the decision to switch off a machine which is sustaining the respiration of a brain-damaged patient. This may arise as a result of a patient being admitted to a casualty department with severe head injuries. He may be given immediate life support from a respirator in order to allow diagnostic and remedial action to be taken. Investigation may then reveal brain damage so extensive, that cerebral death ('irreversible brain damage incompatible with the recovery of consciousness') (Woodruff, 1970, p. 16) is diagnosed. In this situation, assuming that every precaution has been taken to obtain a reliable estimate of the damage, switching off the machine can be regarded as the *abandonment of an attempt to restore life*, since it has become clear that the process of dying cannot be reversed (although it might be arrested for an indefinite period). Removal of the support of the machine permits the process of dying to continue, if the patient is incapable of sustaining respiration spontaneously.

For this reason, the action of switching off the machine can be regarded as permitting death rather than actively causing it. There is no way back to life as normally understood and no benefit to the patient in remaining indefinitely in a state of suspended dying. Critical to this argument is agreement that cerebral death is equivalent to the end of personal existence. This must be the only reason for switching off. Arguments that the machine could be more profitably used for another patient or that the patient on the machine might be an organ donor take on a sinister appearance, if in any sense the body is also still a person.

## Ethical Considerations

The basic moral question underlying all these examples of permitting death is whether they constitute transgression of the medical commitment to respect human life. Some moralists have tried to answer this by drawing a distinction between ordinary and extraordinary means of treatment (*see* Chapter Four, p. 98 *et seq*.). The difficulty with this distinction is that it appears to focus on the method of treatment rather than the condition of the patient. Use of antibiotics, for example, is by now a standard, ordinary means of treatment. Does this entail an obligation to use them even on patients who are very close to death from other more painful conditions? Haemodialysis, on the other hand, is still in the category of the expensive and 'extraordinary'. Yet there would seem to be a pressing obligation to use it, if available, in the case of a young patient. However, some definitions of the distinction relate it to what is 'burdensome' to the patient, rather than to types of treatment. Such an interpretation, in effect, leaves entirely to the discretion of the doctor what treatments to institute or discontinue on the basis of his judgment of 'burdensome'.

How then should the doctor decide? It would appear that all he can do, is to help the patient's dying be as near as possible to what he believes the patient would want. This involves him in awareness of the patient as an individual with certain attitudes, aspirations and beliefs. Some patients may want to 'fight it out' to the last, others may want to 'slip away' as quickly as possible. (The kind of knowledge of the patient which is required is frequently not available to the hospital specialist, who may be seeing the patient for the first time. Since nearly half of all deaths in Britain take place in hospital, implementation of the ideal of personal communication at the time of death requires a health service in which family doctors are involved in hospital as well as home care of their patients.)

When the patient is unconscious or virtually decerebrate the doctor may still feel it right to respect his wishes. He can safely assume that few people want indignity in death or want to prolong distress for their relatives. These assumptions about how the patient would regard what was being done to his body also affect the question of the use of 'heart beat cadavers' for transplantation. If this is largely abhorrent to ordinary people, then there are strong indications against it, at least until lay attitudes re-align themselves with clinical knowledge.

The line of this argument, however, leads us from passive to active euthanasia. If the doctor should avoid what is burdensome to the patient and should respect his wishes, what is he to do if he knows that the patient wants to die more quickly than is likely in the natural course of the illness? May he hasten his death? This question can be approached through discussion of the relief of pain by morphia or other opiates.

### PAIN KILLING AND KILLING

The administration of opiates to patients in order to control pain may hasten death because of the suppressive effect on the respiratory system. Is this then a case of killing the patient rather than merely permitting death to take place? Provided the dosage is commensurate with the degree of pain and is not suddenly increased when the patient's hopeless condition is known, a case can be made out for calling it 'indirect' killing. The argument from 'double effect' (*see* Chapter Four, p. 100 *et seq*.) identifies the *intended* effect to be relief of pain, the merely *allowed* effect to be shortening of life. If the doctor directly intended to bring about death, he would use more rapid and effective means to do so. This argument, however, cannot entirely evade the fact that the doctor must know perfectly well that a likely consequence of increase of dosage is death of the patient. Since he knows, he must bear responsibility for it. [Some writers have pointed out that the use of life-shortening drugs may not be necessary in order to relieve pain (*see* Trowell, 1971; Twycross, 1975). But there are still some instances in which lethal consequences from pain relief seem highly likely.] If then, a doctor is prepared to accept responsibility for shortening life in the course of alleviating suffering, why should he not alleviate suffering by administration of a lethal dose, if this seems the only merciful solution?

## Causing Death

The direct and deliberate killing of a suffering person in order to end his suffering is what is meant by the term 'active euthanasia'. If it is at the request of the person killed it is voluntary euthanasia: if not at his request, it is imposed euthanasia. Only voluntary euthanasia has been seriously debated in recent times and we shall, therefore, concentrate on it.

The Voluntary Euthanasia Bill introduced by Lord Raglan in the House of Lords in 1969 proposed to 'authorise physicians to give euthanasia to a patient who is thought on reasonable grounds to be suffering from an irremediable physical condition of a distressing character, and who has, not less than 30 days previously, made a declaration requesting the administration of euthanasia in certain specified circumstances one or more of which has eventuated'. (*Explanatory Memorandum on the Voluntary Euthanasia Bill*, in Downing, 1969, p. 197. The Bill was defeated at the Second Reading by 61 votes to 40.)

No further argument *for* such a proposal will be added at this point, since the reasons given for it follow from the discussion of the implications of passive euthanasia. It is a proposal which extends the notion of ensuring a good death to cover 'irremediable conditions' (not necessarily terminal ones), and which makes it legal for doctors to kill patients on request (after certification and a lapse of at least 30 days after the request). What arguments can be used *against* such a proposal?

Firstly, it can be opposed on philosophical and legal grounds, in terms of the distinction between *causing* harm and *permitting* harm to occur. This distinction has been carefully and clearly discussed by George P. Fletcher (Fletcher, G. P., 1969), who, writing as a professor of law, is concerned to encourage a more sensitive interpretation of the law as it stands. He argues that killing a patient, say, by injecting air into his veins, can be seen to be an example of an *act* which contravenes the law against homicide. Failure to preserve life, however, can be regarded as an *omission,* which may or may not carry criminal liability depending on the circumstances in which the omission took place and the nature of the relationship between doctor and patient. Since the patient may be shown to expect the doctor not to take unnecessary steps to maintain his life, the doctor's omission of treatment may not be culpable. Whatever the patient's expectations or requests, however, the law cannot sanction *direct causing* of harm to another. (The patient's request for euthanasia does not excuse it from culpability.) Similar points have been made by Meyers (1970, Chap. 6). After discussion of the legal sanctions against euthanasia in various countries, he suggests that the law should not affirmatively sponsor killing. It might, however, allow request of the victim or mercy motive of the killer as pleas for mitigation, especially if the killing were carried out within the context of medical care.

Secondly, numerous practical objections to legislation for voluntary active euthanasia have been put forward. The main problems are: ensuring that the request is valid; ascertaining that conditions are fulfilled for certification of 'irremediable conditions'; the avoidance of additional suffering to the patient through the delay required to allow him to change his mind; and the unfortunate grief effects on relatives which 'deaths from euthanasia' might have. (*See* Gould, 1971 for a discussion of all of these.) Defenders of such legislation are theoretically correct in protesting that practical difficulties do not disprove the rightness of the principle. Nevertheless, it remains to be shown how such a principle can be given workable legislative expression. (The proposer of the Bill has since commented that some of the practical difficulties in framing legislation appear 'insuperable'. Raglan, 1972.)

Thirdly, the most fundamental objection to the legalising of euthanasia is its implications for the relationship between patients and their doctors and nurses. The doctor would be authorised to kill patients or to prescribe a lethal dose which may be administered by a nurse. Of course no doctor or nurse could be compelled to do this: the law would merely allow it. Nevertheless, mercy-killing would be defined by law as a valid part of the professional function of doctors and nurses. This in itself would change the character of the relationship with patients, unless the professions opted out as a body from any legislation. (In a recent report, the BMA has declared its opposition to active euthanasia.) The involvement of the two professions in certification of suitable candidates and in administration of euthanasia would appear to cut right across the usual emotional investment of those involved in caring for patients, as well as the normal framework of expectation within which a patient entrusts himself to medical care. In particular, the patient after certification would be in a totally different relationship to his medical attendants. He becomes a person soon to be killed: one of their professions becomes a destroyer of life. (Advocates of euthanasia prefer the phrase, 'abettor of suicide', but this does not accurately describe the positive action the doctor would be required to take.)

A solution to this difficulty might be to appoint and train professional euthanasists. (This was proposed in a 1936 Bill.) But many of the same problems would remain. Doctors would still have to certify suitable candidates, and at the appointed time, the staff caring for a patient would find themselves handing over responsibility to the professional mercy-killer.

The alternative to positive legislation for voluntary euthanasia is the (apparently) less rational and less equitable approach of leaving descisions in each case to be determined by the concern of doctors and nurses to shield patients from suffering and indignity. A guide to students and practitioners in medical ethics contains the following advice by a physician concerning 'acceleration of death in the dying': 'In the first place the law forbids in theory but ignores in practice, thus tacitly accepting the common sense view that doctors here, as in other spheres, should be protected from the consequences of steps honestly taken in the interests of patients.... If there are occasions when hastening death seems the most sensible and humane procedure, the proper course then becomes a matter for one's own conscience, a guide to conduct is found by regarding the circumstances as affecting a close personal relative'. (I. Clifford Hoyle in Davidson, 1957, p. 138).

## Ethics and Euthanasia

In considering the mercy killing of patients, the spheres of law and morality must be distinguished, although it is evident that to some extent they overlap. We have already noted that as the law stands at present direct destruction of the life of a patient, whether or not he has requested it, is murder; and failure to institute life-saving measures might—depending on the circumstances—constitute culpable negligence. Euthanasia legislation would remove certain instances of direct killing of patients from the category of murder. (Failure to carry out treatment would presumably continue to be assessed according to circumstances.)

Whether or not active euthanasia became legal, however, some points of view in ethics would regard it as always morally wrong. Theories which identify a moral law prohibiting 'killing of the innocent' (but not judicial killing of murderers or killing in a 'just war') place mercy killing in the same moral category as murder. Thus Welty (1963, p. 130) states: '... no-one may ask for it, demand, order, suggest it or carry it out; it must be resolutely refused to the sick person (and his relatives), however intense his suffering, however small his hope of recovery.' (Welty goes on to defend this absolute opposition to euthanasia with the argument that: 'It is not God's will, and is neither permitted to us mortals nor indeed possible for us, to strip death of all its terror and pain; death is meant to be the last and greatest test we have to undergo here on earth.')

At the opposite end of the spectrum, the most consistent versions of greatest happiness theory can raise no objection to ending lives which are of no use either to the individual or to society. Provided euthanasia were carefully controlled so that only really hopeless cases were included, social benefit would accrue from painlessly killing not only those with severe pain in terminal illness, but also the grossly deformed and the severely subnormal. Such euthanasia would have to be imposed in cases where consent could not be obtained, but, for the sake of maximising happiness and avoiding pain, this might be regarded as a praiseworthy act of mercy.

Between these two opposing attitudes, a shifting middle ground is occupied both by advocates of *voluntary* euthanasia and by those who, whilst preferring to retain legal sanctions against it, believe that in some instances a physician's conscience may lead him to disregard the law. The assumption shared by both of these approaches to the problem is that the integrity of persons may be more important than the sanctity of human life. The more 'conservative' of the two approaches allows direct attack on life only in exceptional circumstances, when all other measures to prevent suffering have failed. The more 'liberal' view believes that each person has a right to decide for himself that his life should be ended, if certain irremediable medical conditions ensue.

If such a middle ground is sought, there are no simple answers to the euthanasia question. The choice would appear to be between the uncertainty of the present legal situation in which a patient's trust might be betrayed by too little, or too much, action by his doctor and in which a doctor may be forced to risk prosecution out of concern for his patient; and, on the other hand, the cold logic of a law which would formalise a situation whose essentials are trust and sensitivity to another's need. There is no doubting the awareness of suffering which motivates proposals for voluntary euthanasia. The problem is finding appropriate structures through which the rational and emotional aspects of compassion can be given expression.

It is at this point of the argument that moral law theory appears to come into its own. Advocates for voluntary euthanasia legislation seem to underrate the exemplary character of the law. Much has been said earlier about the inflexible character of the legalist approach to morality (see Chapter Three), but the protective function of law should also be acknowledged. A legal system which enshrines the inviolability of human life (including the lives of those found guilty of murder) may appear to dispense rough justice to people who kill others with the best of motives. But the justice would be much rougher in a situation in which killing became legal. The burden of proof would then shift to the state to prove that a given instance of 'voluntary euthanasia' was a violation of law. For this reason the argument of natural law theorists that some moral rules have an absoluteness which protects human values carries considerable weight. It should be noted, however, that 'rule-utilitarianism' would draw a similar conclusion. Arguing from the standpoint of the security afforded to the majority by consistent laws against killing, it would acknowledge that in some instances the unhappiness of a minority may have to be accepted.

In any case, it often seems that intolerable distress and suffering in some terminal conditions have been too easily regarded as inevitable. A positive outcome of the campaign for voluntary euthanasia has been increased concern about developing new facilities for care of the dying and new techniques for relief of pain (Saunders, 1960; Twy-cross, 1975).

## Human Experimentation

The subject of human experimentation carries with it for many people the overtones of Nazi concentration camps. Moreover, recent literature on the topic reveals serious issues of consent and of justifiable risk in relation to some current research projects (Pappworth, 1967; Barber, 1973). Yet advances in medical care depend to a considerable extent on the refinement and expansion of scientific research in all areas of knowledge relevant to the normal functioning of the human body and the overcoming of disease. An indispensable part of such research is the study of human subjects, including those suffering from illness or disability. These may seem statements of the obvious, but it is important that they should be remembered and given proper weight in any discussion of the ethical issues in research involving patients. Focusing attention on cases in which moral problems are evident may give a misleading picture of medical research as a whole, the necessity and propriety of which seems to be beyond question in the vast majority of instances (*see* Rosenheim, 1967; Beecher, 1970).

Much research in medicine is based on the detailed clinical examination of patients, including the use of investigative techniques, such as x-ray photography, biopsy, ECG and EEG monitoring. These may raise problems, if there is discomfort or risk disproportionate to the patient's potential benefit. If however the examination is clearly necessary in order to make an accurate diagnosis, there seems to be no moral objection to using the information gathered in research, provided confidentiality is respected.

*Experimentation* proper may be defined as '... the conscious manipulation of the patient's clinical situation, altering some aspect of his management to gather information, answer some specific question or devise a new treatment' (Pellegrino, 1969, p. 34). Such experimentation may be of direct benefit to the patient (e.g. trying out a new drug or new operative technique); of indirect benefit to the patient (e.g. studies of physiological processes whose relationship to the patient's disease is being investigated); or of no benefit to the patient (studies of processes or drugs of no known relevance to his disease). The third category of experimentation is really outside the area of clinical care and includes the use of normal volunteer subjects either as experimental subjects or as control subjects.

The World Medical Association has drawn up a code of ethics for human experimentation which makes a fundamental distinction between research in which 'the aim is essentially therapeutic for a patient', and research 'the essential object of which is purely scientific and without therapeutic value to the person subjected to the research' (*Declaration of Helsinki*, 1964). This distinction will provide the framework for our discussion of ethical issues in experimentation, although some examples of research seem to fall partly into each category.

## NON-THERAPEUTIC RESEARCH

'In the purely scientific application of clinical research carried out on a human being it is the duty of the doctor to remain the protector of the life and health of that person on whom clinical research is being carried out' (*Declaration of Helsinki*, Section 3, clause 1).

The use of human beings as experimental material to gain information which will be of no direct benefit to them raises two fundamental questions: the degree of anxiety, discomfort or physical risk which it is permissible to impose on subjects; and the nature of the consent obtained for participation in the experiment. These issues are raised sharply by a research project carried out in Willowbrook Residential School for mentally subnormal children in Staten Island, New York (see Goldman, 1971; New York University School of Medicine, 1973). In this project, which was set up in 1956 to study viral hepatitis and to try to discover an effective vaccine against it, selected groups of new admissions to the school were admitted to a special experimental unit in which they were deliberately infected with the disease. The experimenters justified this procedure on the grounds that, since the disease was rife in the institution anyway, the children were almost bound to get it sooner or later. By being infected under controlled conditions, it was argued, they would be less at risk and would be cared for in ideal circumstances. The objectionable aspect of this experiment was that it involved deliberately causing distress to children who could not understand what was happening to them. Moreover, it was not inevitable that these children would get the disease. This was inevitable only if nothing were done to reduce the incidence of the disease in the institution as a whole through methods of treatment and control known at the time. Thus the gaining of consent from parents for use of the children involved using the incidence of the diseases as a way of coercing co-operation. We shall now consider in turn the factors of *risk* to the subject and of *valid consent*, which this case illustrates.

*Risk*

Like any term assigning value to human interaction the notion of justifiable risk is open to wide interpretation. As Pappworth (1967, p. 13) points out: 'What may appear relatively innocuous to the hardened experimenter can produce extreme distress, including a good deal of fear in a patient who is being submitted to something he does not understand properly'. It seems essential to include the causing of psychological distress in any reckoning of risks involved, even although it may be argued that no permanent damage will be caused. For this reason (and others given in the next section) the use of children in experiments of no direct benefit to them is open to question. In the case of adult volunteers, the general principle of protecting the health of the subject means that experiments should not be carried out when there is the possibility of permanent damage to subjects, or when the possible effects are difficult to assess accurately. Uncertainty over these matters would indicate that more animal experimentation should be carried out before human subjects are used.

The objective assessment of risk seems to require the examination of research proposals by qualified persons other than the experimenter himself. In Britain at the present time many hospitals and research establishments have research committees to discuss the scientific and ethical aspects of research proposals, but there is no statutory requirement for such bodies nor any system for centralised reporting and control of experiments. Opinions vary as to whether a line of control should be established through the General Medical Council and the Ministry of Health (Pappworth, 1967, p. 208f.), or whether clinical investigation should be free to proceed without 'unnecessary interference and delay' and without the '... imposition of rigid or central bureaucratic controls' (Rosenheim, 1967). (For a full discussion of procedures and controls in clinical research *see* Barber *et al.*, 1973; Katz, 1972; May, 1975.)

## Valid Consent

Assuming that subjects are not being asked to undergo undue risk or discomfort, the manner in which their co-operation is enlisted is also important. In non-therapeutic research the subject has no need to participate in order to benefit his own health. For this reason, the obtaining of *valid consent* is essential. This may be defined as 'the freely given consent of the fully informed subject'.

In an earlier discussion of responsibility (*see* Chapter Five) two factors necessary for voluntary decision were noted: absence of coercion, and knowledge of the consequences of the actions contemplated. This means that valid consent is obtained only if the subject it told everything that is involved in the experiment and *is able to understand what is being explained*, and if he is under no constraint to agree to take part. If these criteria are strictly applied, whole classes of potential subjects are automatically ruled out from participation in non-therapeutic research. On grounds of inability to understand what is involved, one must exclude children, the mentally subnormal, the psychiatrically ill (in some instances), the elderly, and confused, and any patient whose ability to think clearly is affected by illness. On grounds of constraint, any one in a dependent relationship to the researcher might be excluded—for example, a clinician's own patients or a clinical teacher's students.

How scrupulous should a researcher be in ensuring that he has obtained a valid consent? In terms of law in Britain at least, it is unlikely that a parent is entitled to give consent to procedures of no benefit to his children, although this principle has never been tested in court (Meyers, 1970, Chap. 4). In general, however, the legal controls in most countries are limited to those broad rules which prevent negligence and malpractice in medical care. Much is left to the humanity and good judgment of the researcher himself. These qualities are under the greatest test when the researcher is deciding what is meant by the 'fully informed' subject. Taking blood samples, for example, carries a slight risk of infection, but one which the researcher may regard as minimal. He may often decide not to alarm subjects unnecessarily by describing unlikely risks, contenting himself with a simple request to take a blood sample, and an explanation of why it is needed. On the other hand, the use of cardiac catheterisation to obtain samples, without telling subjects that this procedure will be involved (*see* Pappworth, 1967, p. 193) illustrates that the desire not to cause alarm may lead to actively misleading patients about what it is they are consenting to.

### THERAPEUTIC RESEARCH

'In the treatment of the sick person the doctor must be free to use a new therapeutic measure if in his judgment it offers hope of saving life, re-establishing health, or alleviating suffering (*Declaration of Helsinki*, Section 2, clause 1).

The focus of attention shifts significantly when one moves from research of no direct benefit to the patient to investigations or clinical experiments which may alleviate his condition. In this situation, the critical judgment to be made concerns the relative balance of risk and benefit. An extreme example will demonstrate this. In the early 1950's medical scientists began to accumulate evidence that the treatment of premature infants with high concentrations of oxygen was causing retrolental fibroplasia, a condition leading to blindness. Three American doctors set up an experiment to prove that this was the case by giving 36 premature infants high concentrations of oxygen for two weeks. (A control group of 28 infants was given low concentrations.) The experiment established the connection, but at the cost of permanent blindness for eight of the subjects (Lanman *et al.*, 1954). It could be argued that this was 'therapeutic research', in the sense that it was investigating a disease which all the experimental subjects might have developed. But, in view of what was already suspected about the damaging effects of oxygen, the risk far outweighed the potential benefit.

The issue of valid consent is also important in therapeutic research, as it is in all medical interventions in a patient's life. In some instances it may be necessary to proceed without consulting the patient, either because he is too ill to exercise choice, or because fully informing him of the balance of risks might be detrimental to his recovery. In such situations the doctor can be regarded as acting *for* the patient, taking a decision as though he were the patient. This may be of particular importance when treatment of dying patients is being contemplated. In these circumstances measures might be tried which would never be used were the condition of the patient not already hopeless. (Given the opportunity to choose, a patient *might* be glad to be used to test out an uncertain therapeutic measure, in the hope that it may help others if not himself, but in a great many cases there is no way of knowing what the patient would wish.)

## Organ Transplantation

A number of specific issues are raised by organ transplantation which merit separate discussion. Some of these issues relate back to the preceding section, providing further illustration of the dilemmas of clinical research: others relate specifically to the organ donor.

For practical purposes, discussion can be limited to kidney and heart transplantation, since these are the organs most commonly transplanted into human recipients at present. Moreover, of these two types of transplantation, only replacement of a kidney can yet be regarded as a properly established treatment measure. In the case of kidney transplantation, three types of human donor have been used: living related donors, living unrelated donors and cadaver (normally unrelated) donors. Heart transplantation allows, in the nature of the case, only cadaver donors. In both areas of transplantation some attempts to use animal donors have been made, but rejection problems are so great that there seems no immediate prospect of successful transplantation from this source (Woodruff, 1970, p. 24). Artificial organs, most likely the artificial heart in the first instance, may in the future be ingrafted, again if incompatibility problems can be overcome.

So far as moral dilemmas are concerned, separate issues arise as regards the recipient and as regards the donor.

### THE RECIPIENT

Is the risk and discomfort attendant upon organ transplantation justifiable? The first point to be remembered is that, without such major surgery, the recipient is faced with the likelihood of death from failure of a vital organ. Thus the risks of intervention have to be balanced against the risks of non-intervention. The situation in the case of renal failure is alleviated by the possibility of haemodialysis as an alternative line of treatment, but this has its own problems, both physical and psychological, and alleviates rather than cures the condition. (In many cases the use of one or more renal transplant in conjunction with intermittent dialysis proves the most satisfactory treatment measure.) The serious illness of a patient, however, does not justify *any* procedure. As has already been argued, the use of experimental methods of treatment with a low chance of success may do no more than add to the patient's suffering. In transplantation both the effect of surgery itself and the possibly adverse side-effects of immuno-suppressive drugs have to be reckoned with. What has to be decided is whether the patient is being offered a reasonable chance of survival and freedom from disability.

What is a 'reasonable chance'? This is the crux of the difficulty. It is a simple matter to set an ideal, toward which transplantation is aiming. This would be to give the recipient the same life expectancy as a person of the same age, whose heart or kidney was functioning normally. (One must allow for the fact that many recipients will have other disorders which will continue as a threat to life, however successful the transplantation.) Heart transplantation and kidney transplantation in their early stages have fallen far short of this ideal. [In the period December 1967 to June 1970, 160 heart transplants had been carried out, but only 10 recipients survived (*see* Smith, 1970, p. 102). The 1963 statistics for kidney transplants showed a survival rate of 84 per cent of recipients of identical twin kidneys after one year: but only 11 per cent of recipients of related donor kidneys and 2 per cent of recipients of cadaver donors (*see* Woodruff, 1964).] The other side of the picture, however, is the steady improvement in success rates for renal transplantation, as difficulties of tissue matching and rejection of the graft have diminished. One year survival rates for unrelated donors as high as 95 per cent have been reported, and it has been estimated that more that half of all recipients, since transplantation began in the early 1950's, still survive (Lyons, 1970, p. 40). In these figures for renal transplantation, results appear to be approaching the reasonable. Such progress might not have been achieved without earlier work, in which the success rates were much lower.

Thus the dilemma of all clinical experimental procedures presents itself: the choice is between not carrying out too risky a procedure, and advancing a technique which will benefit sufferers from the same disease in the future. The points made in the previous section, seem relevant to this dilemma: Provided patients are allowed to be participators in the decision, there appears to be no moral objection and considerable potential moral worth in asking them to undergo surgery after they have been fully informed of the options open to them. Moral boundaries would be crossed if patients (or those giving consent on their behalf) were given inadequate information or misled about the likelihood of success.

Some particular points relate specifically to transplantation. (1) In heart transplantation the absence of the 'safety net' which dialysis provides for kidney transplantation makes the risks much higher. In view of the low success rate, it may be seen as an unwarranted surgical procedure which should not be offered to patients until rejection problems show some solution in animal experiments, or until a back-up procedure equivalent to haemodialysis is available. (2) A dilemma will persist in the potential use of grafts from animals or in the use of artificial organs. These would not raise the same donor problems as grafts from humans, but, so long as the human source is the more reliable, it seems wrong for a surgeon not to use human donors. (3) If patients are in a badly deteriorated state (*see* for example, the description of the recipient of the chimpanzee's heart in Hardy, 1964), it is questionable whether surgery is justifiable. In such cases the patient appears to have been reduced to a means for testing a technique.

## THE DONOR

Separate problems arise in the case of living donors and cadaver donors. In renal transplantation the best results have been obtained by using kidneys from related donors, virtually perfect compatibility being obtained in the case of identical twins. The use of any living donor means that a healthy person is being subjected to risk both from the operation itself and from the possibility that his remaining kidney might fail at some future date. From some points of view an operation of this kind can be described as 'mutilation' or 'maiming' (Bentley, 1966), since it entails the removal of a part of the body to no benefit to the well-being of the body as a whole. However, the risk that the donor's other kidney might fail has been estimated at 0·07 per cent, whilst post-operative risk has been estimated at 0·05 per cent (Hamburger, 1966). If these estimates are accurate, the term 'maiming' may seem somewhat over-dramatic, even if theoretically correct. It does not seem unreasonable for a person to allow 'maiming' to this extent, if it can save the life of another.

A more serious problem in the use of living donors relates to the concept of valid consent, particularly since the best results are obtained from related donors. Professor G. E. Schreiner has commented: '... do you really believe that any relative watching a uraemic patient die can really give true voluntary consent, i.e., with the absence of coercion?' (Schreiner, 1966). The dangers of pressures from within the donor or from the donor's family have alerted surgeons to the need for careful screening of 'volunteers'. (The right of the hospital to turn down donors on health grounds allows offers to be refused without the donor feeling that he has failed the recipient.)

The problems involved in the use of living donors are largely avoided by the use of cadavers. Consent is less of a moral problem, but, because of the need to remove the organ as soon as possible after death, some difficulties remain. Frequently cadaver donors are accident victims whose relatives have to be approached in distressing circumstances. A solution to this problem would be to encourage people willing to be donors to have their names entered on a central register and carry a card indicating their willingness. An alternative proposal would be to allow organs to be removed unless the donor had expressly indicated his unwillingness. This would be a much looser use of the concept of consent (*see* British Transplantation Society, 1975).

A second area of difficulty centres round the diagnosis of death in the case of cadaver donors. The basic principle has been acknowledged by the World Medical Association that the doctors certifying death must be independent of the transplant team. Because of the time factor involved, however, there must be some communication between them. [Kidneys must be removed in less than one hour, preferably less than 30 minutes. The time lapse possible for heart and liver is even shorter (Woodruff, 1970).] If a patient is on a respirator and seems a suitable candidate for transplantation, may the doctors caring for him delay switching off the machine? Is it permissible to transfer a patient on a respirator from one hospital to another in order to be near the recipient?

Answers to these questions depend on decisions about the time of death of the patient. Moving a still living patient to another hospital simply to assist transplantation would be ethically unacceptable (*see* BMA, 1970), so would prolonging the act of dying in order to keep organs undamaged. But if some patients on respirators are to be regarded as *already dead*, although still possessing some biological functioning, then these actions are not instances of maltreatment of patients. In such a case, some surgeons (e.g. in France and in the USA) may be prepared to go a step further and remove organs *before* circulation has stopped. Clearly, these examples call for a re-appraisal of the diagnosis of death.

As Pope Pius XII wisely remarked, the definition of death is a matter for clinicians not medical laymen (Pius XII, 1957). This is ever more the case as methods for supporting life become more efficient. The layman thinks of death as an *event*, evidenced by the cessation of respiration and heartbeat, but to the clinician it is more accurately described as an irreversible process. Difficulties arise when definitions of death are proposed which allow a person to be diagnosed as dead even when some of the signs, which the layman would regard as signs of life, are still present. Thus recent French legislation allows cerebral death (assessed by a flat EEG reading) to be a sufficient ground for diagnosing 'clinical death' (Meyers, 1970, p. 113). This contrasts quite sharply with the statement of the World Medical Association regarding the determination of the point of death (*Declaration of Sydney*, 1968):

'This determination will be based on clinical judgment supplemented if necessary by a number of diagnostic aids (of which the electroencephalograph is currently the most helpful). However, no single technological criterion is entirely satisfactory in the present state of medicine ...'

Comprehensive definitions of death would regard the irreversible cessation of spontaneous respiration and heart beat as part of the definition of death, to be taken in conjunction with evidence of total absence of cerebral function. But can the circulatory system be exempted from the necessary conditions, provided cerebral death is evidenced by a series of tests (see e.g. G. P. J. Alexandre's test in Wolstenholme, 1966, p. 69)? If so, then is the use of 'heart beat cadavers' in transplantation justifiable?

There are two separate answers to this question. One is an answer in terms of reliability of diagnosis, and this can be decided by medical opinion. But a second answer needs to be found in terms of the non-medical public's understanding of death. It seems possible that the patient may not want to be a 'heart beat cadaver', from whom organs are removed. He may want to be sure he has 'died properly', as he understands it, before being regarded as a donor. Yet has he the right to be so scrupulous at the expense of the lives of others?

### ETHICS AND PRIORITIES

If we compare arguments about organ transplantation with arguments about medical research, we come upon some interesting contrasts. Proponents for transplantation tend to lay stress on the benefit accruing to the particular patients who need such life-saving measures: defenders of unfettered clinical research more commonly emphasise the benefits to humanity of advances in medical science. Those who have hesitations about transplant surgery question the justification of high cost procedures which benefit only a few: those who are concerned about aspects of clinical research focus on infringement of the rights of individuals in the name of community benefit. Pellegrino (1969, p. 32) has clearly described this contrast as it relates to the doctor–patient relationship:

The patient-subject and physician-helper dichotomies are an irremediable complexity of human experimentation and the distinctions between them must not be blurred out ... Individual good is necessarily counterposed against the common good; scientific values are placed against personal and human values; and, even the rights of future generations are potentially compromised by the rights of those living today. The expectations of society can only be fulfilled by a critical ordering of these conflicting values in such a way that experimentation on humans can be used to advance the good of man without violating his humanity in the process.

The 'critical ordering of conflicting values' in an issue of this kind could be regarded as a final testing ground for the ethical theories we have surveyed. We see in the struggles of John Stuart Mill to be both humane and consistently utilitarian one attempt to do justice to both individual and societal values. For Mill this meant building in certain 'end stops' to the greatest happiness calculation. Liberty, truth, beauty were never to be taken away from individuals in the name of some higher social good. These sentiments sound admirable, yet Mill's ideals can easily degenerate into a defence of an individualism which is blind to social and political realities. It was the rough arithmetic of Bentham which pinpointed the social inequalities of his time. It might be argued that an effective preparation for discussions of the quality of life which medical science offers would be first to subject the statistics of world medical facilities to

Bentham's crude counting of heads. Such an approach would give some indication of how accurate are the claims of medical researchers and surgical pioneers to be benefiting mankind as a whole. It would seem a pity to allow compromises in valid consent if the research turns out after all to have only a tangential connection with social benefit.

For Kantian ethics, of course, calculations of this kind are unnecessary and irrelevant. In view of the certainty of the moral law and the uncertainty of human predictions there should be no compromise with the rights of the individual. All research on subjects incapable of giving full and free consent would have to cease, even if the risk entailed were minimal. All measures to *save* lives would have to be employed, whatever the economic cost. (We have already observed (Chapter Four) that specific recommendations are not easily drawn from Kantian theory. Kant is more interested in the structure of moral argument than in its practical implementation. But it is hard to see what other conclusions could be drawn from a theory which emphasises doing one's duty irrespective of the consequences.) If these are the implications of Kantianism, we can draw little assistance from it for the conflict of priorities in medicine. The problem in the priorities question is that the context of the decision is not a one-to-one relationship. Although it seems correct that a doctor should make the benefit of his individual patient his primary goal, it is the *society* which determines in what circumstances and for what conditions the doctor–patient responsibilities are undertaken (at least when public funds are involved). Conversely, matters of initiation of research and consent procedures are not purely the medical researcher's responsibility. His sense of duty alone cannot weigh the protection of the one against the benefit of the many.

It can be argued then that Kant's stress on the autonomy

of the moral agent invalidates his theory so far as the social issues within medical ethics are concerned. The same would be true of Butler's reliance on the authority of the individual conscience. Too easily such an approach degenerates into an insulation of the practitioner from radical re-assessment of the value of his professional activities. The conscience of the doctor or scientist will, at least in part, reflect the mores of his professional community and 'judgment by one's peers' is a re-enforcement of the basic assumptions of the profession. Butler offers no help to the person puzzled by choices for which his prior experience has no value categories.

It seems that the ethical theories we have analysed leave the basic conflict between individual and society unresolved. Yet there may be, from several of the theories, the beginnings of a satisfactory theory of social ethics. The 'respect for persons' component of Kant's theory seems to provide the kind of check and balance which Mill was searching for in his modified utilitarianism. Putting them together would mean accepting the inevitability of compromise and unpredictability in social planning, but taking as a basic norm the maximising of the personal freedom and responsibility of each individual. If such a synthesis is possible, a further difficulty remains. Both Kantianism and Utilitarianism seem deficient in their descriptions of the goals of morality. Kant's account of moral autonomy entails a radical split between reason and emotion and reduces human relationships to obligations. Utilitarianism, on the other hand, is faced with the impossibility of adequately defining human happiness. A way out of these difficulties may be found by defining moral goals in terms of 'interpersonal communication', a concept which has both rational and emotional components. (For an exposition of this idea *see* Chapter Five.) A goal of this kind sets up an order of priority for planning in health care. Disease would be defined as the destruction of relationship capacities and health as their enhancement. From this starting point, the distribution of health care and the concentration of research effort would need to be assessed according to the criterion of equalisation of opportunity for interpersonal communication.

It would be rash to suppose that the tentative synthesis just outlined can survive criticism any better than the classical theories from which it has been created. It allows us, however, to end our critical analysis of ethical theories with the outlines of a new beginning to the search for moral values in medicine.

## Suggestions for Further Reading

Of the writings discussed in this book, the following provide fairly easy reading: Joseph Butler's *Sermons* (paperback edition, S.P.C.K.), David Hume's *Enquiry into the Nature of Morals* (Oxford University Press paperback), John Stuart Mill's essays, *Utilitarianism* and *On Liberty* (available either in Fontana or Everyman series) and Jean-Paul Sartre's *Existentialism and Humanism* (English translation published by Methuen).

More difficulty may be found with the theories of Hobbes, Spinoza and Kant. Their major writings are: Thomas Hobbes, *Leviathan* (abridged edition published by Fontana); Baruch Spinoza, *Ethics* (Everyman series); and Immanuel Kant, *Critique of Practical Reason* (Longmans). Kant's *Fundamental Principles of the Metaphysic of Ethics* (Longmans) is shorter but hardly less obscure.

Some modern works of fiction may provide material for discussion of the issues raised in this book, for example: F. Dostoievsky, *Crime and Punishment*; A. Huxley, *Brave New World*; A. Camus, *The Outsider*; A. Miller, *The Crucible*. (All published in Penguin editions.)

Ongoing discussion of problems in medical ethics is provided by the *Journal of Medical Ethics*, and other publications of the Society for the Study of Medical Ethics (Tavistock House East, Woburn Walk, London); and by annual bibliographies and the journal, *Hastings Centre Report*, published by the Institute of Society, Ethics and the Life Sciences (623 Warburton Avenue, Hastings-on-Hudson, N.Y. 10706).

# REFERENCES

Agate, J. N. (1972). 'Let Me Go in Peace.' *Contact*, **38** supplement, 28-36.

Alexandre, G. P. J. (1966). In *Ethics and Medical Progress*. Ed. Wolstenholme, G. E. W. London: Churchill.

Barber, Bernard, *et al.* (1973) *Research on Human Subjects: Problems of Social Control in Medical Experimentation*. New York: Russell Sage Foundation.

Beecher, H. K. (1970). *Research and the Individual*. Boston: Little Brown.

Bentley, G. V. (1966). In *Ethics and Medical Progress*. Ed. Wolstenholme, G. E. W., p. 19. London: Churchill.

Bonhoeffer, D. (1955). *Ethics*. Translated by Smith, N. H. London: S.C.M.

British Medical Association (1970). *Medical Ethics* (Pamphlet reprinted from the Members Handbook). London: B.M.A.

British Medical Association (1971). *The Problem of Euthanasia*. A report prepared by a special panel appointed by the Board of Science and Education of the British Medical Association. London: B.M.A.

British Transplantation Society (1975). The Shortage of Organs for Clinical Transplantation: Document for Discussion. *British Medical Journal*, **1**, 251-255.

Ciba Foundation (1973). *Law and Ethics of AID and Embryo Transfer*. North-Holland: Elsevier.

Davidson, M. (1957). *Medical Ethics*. London: Lloyd-Luke.

Downing, A. B. (ed.) (1969). *Euthanasia and the Right to Death*. London: Peter Owen.

Downie, R. S. (1971). *Roles and Values*. London: Methuen.

Dunstan, G. R. (1972). Euthanasia: Clarifying the Issues. *Contact*, **38**, 3-8.

Emery, A. E. H. (ed.) (1973). *Antenatal Detection of Genetic Disease*. Edinburgh: Churchill Livingstone.

Finnis, J. M. (1970). Three Schemes of Regulation. In *The Morality of Abortion*. Ed. Noonan, J. T. Cambridge, Mass: Harvard U.P.

Fletcher, G. P. (1969). Prolonging Life: Some Legal Considerations. In *Euthanasia and the Right to Death*. Ed. Downing, A. B. London: Peter Owen.

Fletcher, J. (1955). *Morals and Medicine*. London: Gollancz.

Fletcher, J. (1967). *Moral Responsibility: Situation Ethics at Work*. London: S.C.M.

Gardner, R. F. R. (1972). *Abortion: The Personal Dilemma*. Exeter: The Paternoster Press.

Gerle, B., Lundén, G. & Sandblom, P. (1960). The Patient with Inoperable Cancer from the Psychiatric and Social Standpoints: A Study of 101 Cases. *Cancer*, **13**, 1206-1217.

Goldman, L. (1971). The Willowbrook Debate. *World Medicine*, Sep. 22, **6**, 26, 17-25.

Gould, J. (ed.) (1971). *Your Death Warrant?* London: Chapman.

Hamburger, J. (1966). In *Ethics and Medical Progress*. Ed. Wolstenholme, G. E. W., p. 19. London: Churchill.

Hamilton, M. (ed.) (1972). *The New Genetics and the Future of Man*. Grand Rapids, Mich.: Eerdmans.

Hardy, J. D., Neely, W. A. & Fabian, L. W. (1964). Heart Transplantation in Man: Developmental Studies and Report of a Case. *Journal of the American Medical Association*, **188**, 1132-1140.

Häring, B. (1974). *Medical Ethics*. Slough: St Paul Publications.

Hinton, J. (1967). *Dying*. London: Penguin.

H.M.S.O. (1974). *Report of the Committee on the Working of the Abortion Act*. London: Cmnd. 5579.

Illich, I. (1974). *Medical Nemesis*. London: Calder and Boyars.

Jones, A. and Bodmer, W. F. (1974). *Our Future Inheritance: Choice or Chance?* London: Oxford U.P.

Katz, J., *et al.* (1972). *Experimentation with Human Beings*. New York: Russell Sage Foundation.

Kelly, W. D. and Friesen, S. R. (1950). Do Cancer Patients Want to be Told? *Surgery*, **27** (June), 822-826.

Kübler-Ross, E. (1969). *On Death and Dying*. London: Macmillan.

Lambourne, R. A. (1973). Towards an Understanding of Medico-Theological Dialogue. In *Religion and Medicine 2*, Ed. Melinsky, M. A. H. London: S.C.M. Press.

Lanman, J. T., Guy, L. P. & Dancis, J. (1954). Retrolental Fibroplasia and Oxygen Therapy. *Journal of the American Medical Association*, **155**, 223-226.

Leach, G. (1970). *The Biocrats*. London: Jonathan Cape.

Lyons, C. (1970). *Organ Transplants: The Moral Issues*. London: S.C.M.

May, W. (1975). Composition and Function of Ethical Committees. *Journal of Medical Ethics*. Vol. 1, No. 1 (March).

Meyers, D. W. (1970). *The Human Body and the Law*. Edinburgh: Edinburgh U.P.

New York University School of Medicine, The Student Council (1973). *Ethical Issues in Human Experimentation: The Case of Willowbrook State Hospital Research*. New York: New York University Medical Centre.

Noonan, J. T. (1970). *The Morality of Abortion*. Cambridge, Mass: Harvard U.P.

Pappworth, M. H. (1967) *Human Guinea Pigs: Experimentation on Man*. London: Routledge and Kegan Paul.

Pellegrino, E. D. (1969). The Necessity, Promise and Dangers of Human Experimentation. In *Experiments with Man*. Ed. Weber, H.-R. Geneva: World Council of Churches.

Pius XI (1930). *Casti Connubii*. Papal Encyclical.

Pius XII (1957). Allocution to Doctors and Students. *Acta Apostolicae Sedis*, Vol. XXXXIX, n. 17-18.

Raglan (1972). The Case for Voluntary Euthanasia. *Contact*, **38** supplement, 9-11.

Ramsey, P. (1970). *Fabricated Man*. New Haven: Yale U.P.

Rosenheim, M. L. (1967). *Supervision of the Ethics of Clinical Investigations in Institutions*. Report of the Committee appointed by the Royal College of Physicians of London. *British Medical Journal*, **3**, 429-430.

Sarvis, B. and Rodman, H. (1973). *The Abortion Controversy*. London and New York: Columbia U.P.

Saunders, C. (1960). *The Care of the Dying*. London: Macmillan.

Schreiner, G. E. (1966). In *Ethics and Medical Progress*. Ed. Wolstenholme, G. E. W. London: Churchill.

Smith, H. L. (1970). *Ethics and the New Medicine*, Nashville: Abingdon Press.

Stark, G. (1973). Spina Bifida and Medical Progress. *Contact*, **43**, 9-14.

Trowell, H. (1971). *The Unfinished Debate on Euthanasia*. London: Institute of Religion and Medicine.

Weber, H.-R. (ed.) (1969). *Experiments with Man*. Geneva: World Council of Churches.

Welty, E. (1963). *A Handbook of Christian Social Ethics*, *II*, Edinburgh: Nelson.

Wilson, M. (1971). *The Hospital—A Place of Truth*. University of Birmingham.

Woodruff, M. F. A. (1964). Ethical Problems in Organ Transplantation. *British Medical Journal*, **1**, 1457-1460.

Woodruff, M. F. A. (1970). *The One and the Many*. London: The Royal Society of Medicine.

World Council of Churches (1969). Report of Christian Medical Commission Second Annual Meeting (mimeographed). Geneva: WCC.

World Medical Association (1964). *Declaration of Helsinki*.

World Medical Association (1968). *Declaration of Sydney*.

# Ethical Codes

## The Hippocratic Oath

I swear by Apollo the healer, invoking all the gods and goddesses to be my witnesses, that I will fulfil this Oath and this written Covenant to the best of my ability and judgment.

I will look upon him who shall have taught me this Art even as one of my own parents. I will share my substance with him, and I will supply his necessities, if he be in need. I will regard his offspring even as my own brethren, and I will teach them this Art, if they would learn it, without fee or covenant. I will impart this Art by precept, by lecture and by every mode of teaching, not only to my own sons but to the sons of him who taught me, and to disciples bound by covenant and oath, according to the Law of Medicine.

The regimen I adopt shall be for the benefit of the patients according to my ability and judgment, and not for their hurt or for any wrong. I will give no deadly drug to any, though it be asked of me, nor will I counsel such, and especially I will not aid a woman to procure abortion. Whatsoever house I enter, there will I go for the benefit of the sick, refraining from all wrongdoing or corruption, and especially from any act of seduction, of male or female, of bond or free. Whatsoever things I see or hear concerning the life of men, in my attendance on the sick or even apart therefrom, which ought not to be noised abroad, I will keep silence thereon, counting such things to be as sacred secrets. Pure and holy will I keep my Life and my Art.

If I fulfil this Oath and confound it not, be it mine to enjoy Life and Art alike, with good repute among all men at all times. If I transgress and violate my oath, may the reverse be my lot.

## The Geneva Convention Code of Medical Ethics
Adopted by the World Medical Association in 1949.

*I solemnly pledge* myself to consecrate my life to the service of humanity;

*I will give* to my teachers the respect and gratitude which
· is their due;

*I will practice* my profession with conscience and dignity;

*The health of my patient* will be my first consideration;

*I will respect* the secrets which are confided in me;

*I will maintain* by all the means in my power, the honour and the noble traditions of the medical profession;

*My colleagues* will be my brothers;

*I will not permit* considerations of religion, nationality, race, party politics or social standing to intervene between my duty and my patient.

*I will maintain* the utmost respect for human life from the time of conception; even under threat. I will not use my medical knowledge contrary to the laws of humanity.

*I make these promises* solemnly, freely and upon my honour.

## The International Code of Nursing Ethics

adopted by the International Council of Nurses in July 1953, was revised as below and adopted by the

Grand   Council   meeting   in   Frankfurt,   Germany,
June 1965.

Nurses minister to the sick, assume responsibility for creating a physical, social and spiritual environment which will be conducive to recovery, and stress the prevention of illness and promotion of health by teaching and example. They render health service to the individual, the family and the community and co-ordinate their services with members of other health professions.

Service to mankind is the primary function of nurses and the reason for the existence of the nursing profession. Need for nursing service is universal. Professional nursing service is based on human need and is therefore unrestricted by considerations of nationality, race, creed, colour, politics or social status.

Inherent in the code is the fundamental concept that the nurse believes in the essential freedoms of mankind and in the preservation of human life. It is important that all nurses be aware of the Red Cross Principles and of their rights and obligations under the terms of the Geneva Conventions of 1949.

The profession recognises that an international code cannot cover in detail all the activities and relationships of nurses, some of which are conditioned by personal philosophies and beliefs.

1. The fundamental responsibility of the nurse is threefold: to conserve life, to alleviate suffering and to promote health.

2. The nurse shall maintain at all times the highest standards of nursing care and of professional conduct.

3. The nurse must not only be well prepared to practise but shall maintain knowledge and skill at a consistently high level.

4. The religious beliefs of a patient shall be respected.

5. Nurses hold in confidence all personal information entrusted to them.

6. Nurses not only recognise the responsibilities but the limitations of their professional functions; do not recommend or give medical treatment without medical orders except in emergencies, and report such action to a physician as soon as possible.

7. The nurse is under an obligation to carry out the physician's orders intelligently and loyally and to refuse to participate in unethical procedures.

8. The nurse sustains confidence in the physician and other members of the health team; incompetence or unethical conduct of associates should be exposed but only to the proper authority.

9. The nurse is entitled to just remuneration and accepts only such compensation as the contract, actual or implied, provides.

10. Nurses do not permit their names to be used in connection with the advertisement of products or with any other forms of self-advertisement.

11. The nurse co-operates with and maintains harmonious relationships with members of other professions and with nursing colleagues.

12. The nurse adheres to standards of personal ethics which reflect credit upon the profession.

13. In personal conduct nurses should not knowingly disregard the accepted pattern of behaviour of the community in which they live and work.

14. The nurse participates and shares responsibility with other citizens and other health professions in promoting efforts to meet the health needs of the public—local, state, national and international.

## Human Experimentation
## Code of Ethics of the World Medical Association

A draft code of ethics on human experimentation drawn up by the World Medical Association was published in the British Medical Journal of 27 October, 1962. The original draft of this was in English. A revised version was accepted as the final draft at the meeting of the World Medical Association in Helsinki in June 1964. The original of this draft was in French, of which the W.M.A.'s English version is printed below. It is to be known as the Declaration of Helsinki.

### DECLARATION OF HELSINKI

It is the mission of the doctor to safeguard the health of the people. His knowledge and conscience are dedicated to the fulfilment of this mission.

The Declaration of Geneva of the World Medical Association binds the doctor with the words, 'The health of my patient will be my first consideration'; and the International Code of Medical Ethics which declares that 'Any act of advice which could weaken physical or mental resistance of a human being may be used only in his interest.'

Because it is essential that the results of laboratory experiments be applied to human beings to further scientific knowledge and to help suffering humanity, the World Medical Association has prepared the following recommendations as a guide to each doctor in clinical research. It must be stressed that the standards as drafted are only a guide to physicians all over the world. Doctors are not relieved from criminal, civil, and ethical responsibilities under the laws of their own countries.

In the field of clinical research a fundamental distinction must be recognised between clinical research in which the aim is essentially therapeutic for a patient, and clinical research the essential object of which is purely scientific and without therapeutic value to the person subjected to the research.

## I *Basic Principles*

1. Clinical research must conform to the moral and scientific principles that justify medical research, and should be based on animal experiments or other scientifically established facts.

2. Clinical research should be conducted only by scientifically qualified persons and under the supervision of a qualified medical man.

3. Clinical research cannot legitimately be carried out unless the importance of the objective is in proportion to the inherent risk to the subject.

4. Every clinical research project should be preceded by careful assessment of inherent risks in comparison to foreseeable benefits to the subject or to others.

5. Special caution should be exercised by the doctor in performing clinical research in which the personality of the subject is liable to be altered by drugs or experimental procedure.

## II *Clinical Research Combined with Professional Care*

1. In the treatment of the sick person the doctor must be free to use a new therapeutic measure if in his judgment it offers hope of saving life, re-establishing health, or alleviating suffering.

If at all possible, consistent with patient psychology, the

doctor should obtain the patient's freely given consent after the patient has been given a full explanation. In case of legal incapacity consent should also be procured from the legal guardian; in case of physical incapacity the permission of the legal guardian replaces that of the patient.

2. The doctor can combine clinical research with professional care, the objective being the acquisition of new medical knowledge, only to the extent that clinical research is justified by its therapeutic value for the patient.

## III *Non-Therapeutic Clinical Research*

1. In the purely scientific application of clinical research carried out on a human being it is the duty of the doctor to remain the protector of the life and health of that person on whom the clinical research is being carried out.

2. The nature, the purpose, and the risk of clinical research must be explained to the subject by the doctor.

3a. Clinical research on a human being cannot be undertaken without his free consent, after he has been fully informed; if he is legally incompetent the consent of the legal guardian should be procured.

3b. The subject of clinical research should be in such a mental, physical, and legal state as to be able to exercise fully his power of choice.

3c. Consent should, as a rule, be obtained in writing. However, the responsibility for clinical research always remains with the research worker; it never falls on the subject, even after consent is obtained.

4a. The investigator must respect the right of each individual to safeguard his personal integrity, especially if the subject is in a dependent relationship to the investigator.

4b. At any time during the course of clinical research the subject or his guardian should be free to withdraw permission for research to be continued. The investigator or the investigating team should discontinue the research if in his or their judgment it may, if continued, be harmful to the individual.

# INDEX

Printed in Hong Kong
by Commonwealth Printing Press Ltd

# Notes

NOTES